Differential Diagnosis Mnemonics

Differential Diagnosis Mnemonics

Thomas J. Donnelly, MD
Pulmonary and Critical Care Consultants
Dayton, Ohio

Christopher C. Giza, MD
Assistant Researcher
Division of Neurosurgery
University of California
Los Angeles, California

HANLEY & BELFUS, INC. / Philadelphia

Publisher   HANLEY & BELFUS, INC.
Medical Publishers
210 South 13th Street
Philadelphia, PA 19107
(215) 546-7293; 800-962-1892
FAX (215) 790-9330
Web site: http://www.hanleyandbelfus.com

Note to the reader: Although the information in this book has been carefully reviewed for correctness of dosage and indications, neither the authors nor the editors nor the publisher can accept any legal responsibility for any errors or omissions that may be made. Neither the publisher nor the editors make any warranty, expressed or implied, with respect to the material contained herein. Before prescribing any drug, the reader must review the manufacturer's current product information (package inserts) for accepted indications, absolute dosage recommendations, and other information pertinent to the safe and effective use of the product described.

Library of Congress Cataloging-in-Publication Data

Donnelly, Thomas J., 1962–
    Differential Diagnosis Mnemonics / Thomas J. Donnelly, Christopher C. Giza.
      p. ; cm.
    Includes bibliographical references and index.
    ISBN 1-56053-311-0 (alk. paper)
     1. Diagnosis, Differential. 2. Mnemonics. I. Giza, Christopher C., 1965–
    II. Title.
    [DNLM: 1. Diagnosis, Differential—Terminology—English. 2. Association
Learning—Terminology—English. WB 15 D685d 2000]
    RC71.5.D66 2001
    616.07'5'014—dc21

                                      99-088120

Differential Diagnosis Mnemonics   ISBN 1-56053-311-0

Last digit is the print number: 9 8 7 6 5 4 3 2 1

CONTENTS

Clinical Conditions or Diagnoses

VII. Nephrology

General Considerations

Clinical Symptoms and Signs

Clinical Conditions or Diagnoses

VIII. Acid-Base

General Considerations

Clinical Conditions and Diagnoses

IX. Gastroenterology

Clinical Symptoms and Signs

PREFACE

Generating a useful and complete differential diagnosis is a keystone of clinical medicine. Many texts exist which provide exhaustive lists of possible diagnoses for a particular complaint. It is refining such lists into useful differentials that is part of the "art" of medicine. Memorizing lists of diagnoses can be a daunting task, and a dry one at that. By using mnemonics as a framework, we wish to make learning differential diagnoses more palatable and even enjoyable. In addition, we present an organizational approach to differential diagnosis that is practical and easily learned. The mnemonics presented here range from concise lists that may be committed to memory after the first read, to more lengthy, comprehensive listings that can be looked up when needed. In almost all cases, the mnemonics themselves spell out something that refers to the symptom or diagnosis, increasing the likelihood of remembering it.

Throughout a student's medical education, he or she receives countless little tips or "pearls" that are of immense practical worth but are often difficult to look up in the typical medical textbook. After each mnemonic, we have included many pearls that refer to the symptom or condition described. Some of these tips are just one-liners; others are small tables or outlines that help organize commonly referenced information.

We hope you find this to be a useful handbook that provides a sound organizational framework for approaching differential diagnoses. The mnemonic format necessarily led to some creative listings, which should be easily remembered as well as amusing. We welcome any suggestions or new mnemonics from our readers.

Tom Donnelly
Chris Giza

I

INTRODUCTION

The purpose of this book is to help medical students and clinicians form comprehensive differential diagnoses for common internal medicine and neurology problems. It is an aid for organizing diagnostic possibilities quickly and effectively in clinical situations.

A number of excellent references provide comprehensive lists of differential diagnoses. This book was created with a similar purpose in mind, but we present an approach based on mnemonics. The mnemonics are intended to provide simple frameworks on which to construct differential diagnoses. They are not intended to be the sole source of information, and primary texts should be read to fully understand disease pathogenesis. It is doubtful that anyone can remember every mnemonic in this book. We hope that those for commonly encountered problems will be retained; the others can be referenced should a particular problem arise.

Most students and residents are familiar with numerous disease processes, but have difficulty giving an exhaustive differential diagnosis from memory for a particular clinical entity. This problem often stems from the lack of an organizational framework. Once differential diagnoses are considered in terms of "categories" of illness, they are much easier to complete. We have attempted to identify a wide variety of clinical scenarios and organize a differential diagnosis for each. Some entities are common, such as anemia or renal failure, while others are more specialized, such as refractory hypotension. Having a complete list of possible diagnoses at the outset will lead to the correct diagnosis even in the most complex cases. This approach encourages thoroughness in evaluations, so that diagnoses are not missed.

The mnemonics range in length depending on the clinical entity. Sometimes more than one has been included for brevity or organizational reasons. The best mnemonics are concise, pertinent words or phrases constructed to reflect the pathogenesis of the problem. Others are no more than simple words that help in remembering a list of possibilities. An explanatory section is included with each mnemonic to review pathogenesis or provide helpful information. Some commonly used mnemonics (authors generally unknown) are included in deference to their history or for lack of a better replacement. Finally, please forgive any "artistic" license taken in the creation of these mnemonics.

How to Use This Book

The chapters are divided by organ system and presented with a common organizational theme. A "General Considerations" section starts some chapters to provide an overview of differential diagnosis and clinical assessment pertinent to that particular system. Specific mnemonics, which are divided into two sections, follow. The first section, "Clinical Symptoms and Signs," lists mnemonics that refer to specific clinical complaints by the patient (e.g., cough, headache), or to particular clinical signs detectable on careful physical examination (e.g., jaundice, ataxia). The second mnemonic section, "Clinical Conditions and Diagnoses," lists differential diagnoses for clinical conditions detected through the use of various diagnostic tests (such as thrombocytopenia, hypernatremia), general mnemonics for broad diagnoses (e.g., sexually transmitted disease, pneumothorax), and specific mnemonics that refer to a particular disorder (such as rheumatoid arthritis, AIDS).

Thus, the first section is intended to help in making a differential diagnosis list based primarily on the chief complaint or a significant clinical sign, after the initial history and physical. The second section is aimed at generating more specific differentials based upon initial diagnostic testing and careful consideration of the overall clinical syndrome. Each section is listed alphabetically for ease of reference.

General Approach to Differential Diagnoses

The differential diagnosis for any medical problem can be thought of in terms of categories of disease. The mnemonic **"MEDICINE DOC"** may be used as a general approach to any patient:

Metabolic disease (e.g., nutritional deficiency, dyslipidemias, porphyria)
Endocrine disease (thyroid disease, diabetes)
Drugs/medicines (iatrogenic, accidental, self-administered)
Infections (e.g., bacterial, viral, fungal, mycobacterial, protozoal, helminthic)
Congenital abnormalities (inherited anatomic, immunologic and metabolic disorders)
Immunologic disease (collagen vascular diseases, asthma, acquired immunodeficiency)
Neoplasms (e.g., primary, metastatic, paraneoplastic)
Exotic ("strange" diseases of unknown etiology such as sarcoid, histiocytosis X)
Degenerative processes (e.g., Alzheimer's, amyotrophic lateral sclerosis)
Occupational/environmental exposures (e.g., asbestos, hypersensitivity, trauma)
Cardiovascular diseases (e.g., arrhythmias, atherosclerosis, pulmonary embolus, congestive heart failure)

This list includes the primary etiologies for most medical problems. There is, of course, some overlap between categories: atherosclerosis is both a cardiovascular and metabolic disease; both infections and collagen vascular diseases may cause cardiovascular disease; many of the "exotic diseases" may have an immunologic basis, and many immunologic diseases are exotic. The redundancy is necessary, however, since some entities are difficult to classify or may be forgotten if a framework based solely on pathogenesis is used. For example, where does one classify arrhythmias or pulmonary embolus? Both are common entities that have many causes. The cardiovascular category helps you to remember these common problems in unusual presentations.

When faced with any clinical problem, you can use either the MEDICINE DOC mnemonic or another, more specific mnemonic to develop a differential diagnosis. For example, if a patient has renal failure, you can construct a differential based on the categories in MEDICINE DOC or use the specific **"I CHASE A RISING BUN,"** which lists specific causes of renal failure:

Pre-renal
Intravascular volume depletion (dehydration, third spacing)
Cardiac causes (CHF, MI, tamponade)
Hepatorenal syndrome
Arterial disease (renal artery stenosis)
Shock
Eclampsia/obstetrical complications
Pre-renal/Renal
Acute tubular necrosis ("ATN" in a sense, both "pre-" and "renal" in etiology)
Renal
Radiographic contrast and other toxins (drugs, rhabdomyolysis, hemolysis)
Intrarenal emboli (cholesterol, DIC)
Scleroderma
Interstitial nephritis
Necrotizing vasculitis (polyarteritis nodosa, Wegener's)
Glomerulonephritis
Post-renal
Bladder obstruction (usually prostatism, sometimes blood, pus, calculi)
Ureteral obstruction (calculi, retroperitoneal fibrosis, cancer)
Necrosis of renal papillae (diabetes, sickle cell anemia, NSAID abuse, infection)

The two approaches provide fairly comprehensive lists of possibilities, and there are strengths and weaknesses for both. MEDICINE DOC allows broad classification of disease processes, while I CHASE A RISING BUN lists specific causes of renal failure and organizes them in pre-renal, renal, and post-renal categories. It is helpful to look at medical problems using both types of approach.

Thinking About Differential Diagnoses

Two thought processes are helpful in approaching differential diagnoses:

1. What is the most likely diagnosis? This "gestalt" approach involves looking at the entire picture first and formulating a hypothesis to explain it. After reviewing all the data for a case, decide which diagnosis is most likely. The thinking process from this point focuses on proving or disproving the hypothesis. This approach is helpful for more simple cases, although most clinicians use it to some extent in all cases. Pay careful attention to any aspects that are inconsistent with the presumptive diagnosis and be able to account for them. **Avoid becoming fixated on a diagnosis and ignoring data that do not support it.**

2. What are the patient's problems? This approach focuses on the "parts" or individual aspects of the case. List all of the patient's problems and consider a differential diagnosis for each. Then, attempt to formulate a unifying diagnosis that explains the data, creating a whole from the parts. This technique is helpful when faced with complex cases featuring multiple symptoms and large amounts of data.

The mnemonic approach to differential diagnosis emphasizes starting with a complete list of possibilities. Certain entities on the list will be very uncommon and unlikely in most circumstances. Common entities are considered in the initial differential diagnosis of a problem, but other aspects of a particular patient's case may direct the work-up to more unusual entities. This approach is appropriate as long as you do not ignore features that may be inconsistent with the presumed diagnosis.

Another approach to defining a long list of diagnostic possibilities is to develop a second or perhaps even a third list based on a second sign or symptom of the patient. If you assume that the manifestations of the disease in question are secondary to one process, then you can limit the number of possibilities by only pursuing diagnoses that are on both lists. Be careful using this approach, because patients may have more than one disease process at work, and important diagnostic considerations may be eliminated prematurely. Again, it is critical to always refer back to the complete list of differential diagnostic possibilities when all the features of a case do not add up to a coherent picture.

Sources of Error in Differential Diagnosis

Decision analysis is a process that attempts to classify errors in medical reasoning, with the goal of improving the accuracy of differential diagnosis and ensuring that a critical diagnosis is not missed. Although controversy exists in applying decision analysis to clinical settings, it is worthwhile to understand the sources of error. One approach focuses on first outlining **the basic steps in arriving at a presumptive diagnosis** and then classifying errors according to where they occur in those basic steps. The basic steps are:

1. **Triggering**—determining a diagnostic possibility based on patient information.

2. **Framing**—establishing the context within which the problem will be solved.
3. **Gathering and processing**—reviewing and interpreting diagnostic data; selecting and discarding possible diagnoses
4. **Verification**—reaching a final diagnosis, the one that best fits all of the data.

Errors occur at each of these steps:

Triggering errors may result from a lack of knowledge and associations. Consider the example of a renal failure patient in whom hypotension develops shortly after beginning dialysis. Some clinicians may consider sepsis or hemorrhage (which are plausible), but most nephrologists would immediately think of a pericardial effusion and tamponade as being much more likely. Triggering is an *associative process* that comes with experience.

Framing errors occur when you do not think broadly enough in considering the cause of a patient's problem. For example, a patient with recurrent abdominal pain secondary to hypercalcemia may undergo an extensive gastrointestinal work-up because the differential diagnosis of abdominal discomfort was not framed broadly enough to include metabolic or systemic disorders. This type of error demonstrates the importance of having a complete list of diagnostic possibilities *prior to* embarking on an extensive work-up. It also shows the value of framing the differential diagnosis in two or more contexts (i.e., MEDICINE DOC and a mnemonic for abdominal pain) and then looking at the "intersection" of the sets. Broad framing and framing in multiple contexts may decrease framing errors.

Gathering and processing errors result from misinterpreting test results, not understanding the sensitivity or specificity of a test, or not knowing a particular disease prevalence or likelihood in a given patient. For example, a slightly elevated urinary catecholamine in a 75-year-old patient with severe hypertension may lead a clinician to pursue a diagnosis of pheochromocytoma, even though this is a rare disease. It is much more likely that the catecholamine result is false positive, and the test probably should not have been ordered in the initial evaluation of this patient. Intrinsic renal disease or renovascular disease should be investigated first in this type of patient before looking for more unusual diagnoses. (See "Other Sources of Diagnostic Error" on the next page for additional discussion of probabilistic thinking.)

Verification errors occur when some data supporting a particular diagnosis are obtained, and the patient is then assumed to have that diagnosis, even when other, contradictory data subsequently become available. Failing to account for all aspects of a case and inappropriately adhering to a presumptive diagnosis results in *premature closure*. Consider a woman with fever, rash, anemia, renal insufficiency, and a positive antinuclear antibody test suggesting the diagnosis of systemic lupus erythematosus (SLE). If this patient also had a heart murmur and a negative double-stranded DNA test, these features are less easily explained by a simple diagnosis of SLE (although not impossible). Presumptive immunosuppressive therapy of this patient for a diagnosis of SLE could be hazardous if the patient really has subacute bacterial endocarditis as the cause of her multiple problems.

There also are **"no-fault" errors**. These occur when the patient's findings are highly atypical for the underlying disease, or the disease is extremely uncommon.

An example of this type of error occurred when a young woman on birth control pills presented with dyspnea, chest pain, and a high-probability V/Q scan. Most clinicians would probably initiate anticoagulation, as was done in this case, given this constellation of findings. Subsequently, however, the patient developed cardiac tamponade due to hemorrhagic pericarditis (her actual problem) and had a prolonged intensive care course as a result of the anticoagulation. An arteriogram demonstrated a congenitally stenosed pulmonary artery subsegment, which explained the high-probability V/Q scan. This type of error is unfortunate but, in some cases, unavoidable. No matter how well we perform our duties, errors will occur. This example points to the fact that *you must continue to be vigilant even when a diagnosis seems assured*. Note that premature closure, although understandable in this case, was to the patient's detriment.

The Importance of Probability in Differential Diagnosis

When evaluating the data as they apply to a list of diagnostic possibilities, it is helpful to consider probabilities. Always question:

1. How common is the disease?
2. How common is the disease in the relevant population, i.e. in the particular patient being evaluated?
3. How common is a particular symptom, sign, or laboratory result in the disease being considered?

As you progress in medical education and gain familiarity with different diseases, these questions become easier to answer. Baye's theorem is a mathematical relationship that can be helpful in assessing the probability of one disease versus another, given a particular finding. Probabilities can be calculated based on Baye's rule, which states that the likelihood of a disease in a patient with a given set of findings can be estimated as the proportion of patients with the same findings who also have the disease. For example, the likelihood of pneumonia in a person with fever, cough, and sputum is estimated by dividing the number of people with fever, cough, sputum, and pneumonia by the number of people with fever, cough, and sputum. The actual mathematical calculation is complex, and there are many criticisms of this type of analytical approach, but a few simple and useful points can be offered:

• **Have a general idea of the prevalence and common symptoms** of a particular disease. For example, a young woman with fever, sweating, anxiety, tachycardia, and hypertension may have a pheochromocytoma, but hyperthyroidism also is possible. The above symptoms are characteristic of both disorders; however, hyperthyroidism is much more likely to be the cause because it is more common. The finding of exophthalmos may be seen in Grave's disease, but would not be characteristic of pheochromocytoma, again pointing toward hyperthyroidism as the more likely cause. An evaluation aimed at hyperthyroidism, while keeping pheochromocytoma "on the back burner," would be appropriate in this instance. Also, in the above setting, you should consider an anxiety disorder (even more common) as a possible cause of the patient's symptoms.

• The more specific a finding is, the more helpful it will be in establishing a list of likely diagnoses. **Select one or two pivotal findings** ("pivots") of a patient's case for consideration of the differential diagnosis. Hypercalcemia, for example, is a good pivot because it has a fairly well-defined list of causes. Clubbing also might be helpful as its list of diagnostic possibilities is rather limited. Entities such as chest pain or fatigue are more problematic because they are nonspecific and can occur in a large number of diseases.

• When considering diagnostic possibilities, it is perhaps best to **compare one symptom or finding (pivot) across multiple diseases**, instead of seeking several symptoms or findings for a single disease. This step-wise limitation of data analysis keeps the probabilities of a specific finding in a specific disease in the forefront. The difficulty of this approach is the lack of specific data for the incidence and prevalence of signs and symptoms in specific diseases. Also, the most probable diagnosis based on one symptom may not be the most likely after all the data are considered. The step-wise consideration of single pivots is meant to enhance, rather than replace, good clinical judgment.

Other Sources of Diagnostic Error

• **Giving equal weight to positive and negative findings.** Often we focus on a positive laboratory test result and pursue a diagnosis based on it. Before giving too much weight to a positive result, pay attention to absent supportive elements. This aspect of probabilistic reasoning often is neglected.

• **Using the first information that comes to mind.** This source of error has been termed the "availability heuristic." An example is the immediate consideration of myocardial infarction as a possible diagnosis when a patient presents with chest pain to the emergency room; pericarditis or pulmonary embolism may not come to mind as readily. These latter diagnoses may not be considered initially, and the evaluation and treatment may be misdirected.

• **Looking for evidence that supports an early working hypothesis and ignoring contradictory data.** An example of this so-called confirmation bias is seeking ischemic changes on the EKG of a patient with chest pain, while ignoring more diffuse changes which may be suggestive of pericarditis.

• **Believing in the chosen course of action and favoring evidence that supports it.** Physicians may become too invested in a diagnosis and continue down the wrong pathway in pursuit because of overconfidence.

Summary of Types of Errors

Triggering errors	Not giving equal weight to
Framing errors	positive and negative findings
Gathering and processing errors	The availability heuristic
Verification errors	Confirmation bias
No-fault errors	Overconfidence/overreliance
Premature closure	on a method or dogma

Ways to Avoid Errors

1. Carefully compile information.
2. Pick one or two "pivots."
3. Have a complete differential diagnosis for each pivot.
4. Have at least a general sense of the prevalence of the disease in a given population and in the relevant population for the patient being considered.
5. Have a general idea of the prevalence of a symptom in a particular disease.
6. Do not discard contradictory data when it becomes available. A careful accounting of unexplained aspects of the case is essential.
7. Pay attention to what is not present, i.e., negative findings.
8. Know that differential diagnosis is an imperfect science: *You are fallible.* The unexpected, unlikely, or atypical may occur.

Presenting and Discussing Cases

A few words are in order regarding case presentation and discussion. Case conferences are invaluable teaching exercises. Learning to present cases in a concise and orderly manner teaches the principles of differential diagnosis. Case presentation emphasizes organization of data. Case discussion employs critical thinking and organization of diagnostic possibilities.

Case Presentation

The key to case presentation is brevity. The traditional "H and P" (history and physical) format is the best framework for discussion. Begin with a chief complaint (why the patient came for medical attention) and then proceed with an organized history and physical exam. The history should be discussed in chronological order to avoid confusion. Patients who have been ill for a long time or have been transferred from another hospital typically have extensive and complex histories. It is the duty of the presenter to avoid overly long discussions of previous work-ups or presumptive diagnoses. Focus on the **essential features** of the case.

Tips on Presentation

- Be brief *and* be thorough. You should be able to present most cases completely in 5 minutes or less. Even the most complex cases can be summarized effectively in a brief presentation.
- Present the case in chronological order.
- Avoid cluttering the history with laboratory results, previous work-ups, or other physicians' presumptive diagnoses.
- Follow the traditional "H and P" format:
  a. Chief complaint
  b. History of present illness

c. Past medical history
  d. Medications
  e. Family history
  f. Social history
  g. Review of systems (brief)
  h. Physical exam
- Focus on pertinent positive *and* negative elements.

It usually is best, for the sake of teaching, to omit laboratory results from the initial presentation. This omission emphasizes the importance of a careful clinical evaluation to guide the ordering of laboratory tests. Sometimes the inclusion of laboratory tests is unavoidable since it may be the reason for admission or referral (e.g., anemia). In most cases, however, it is best to first consider diagnostic possibilities and then analyze appropriately focused diagnostic testing.

Note that a thorough history and physical examination should be performed on every patient, and the presenter should be prepared to provide any information if it is requested. However, an exhaustive list of all negative findings is unnecessary.

Describing a Symptom

When considering the differential diagnosis of a patient's symptom or chief complaint, it is essential to obtain a thorough history and accurately describe the problem. Many complaints, such as chest or abdominal pain, have numerous causes, and a more specific description is required to direct the work-up. Consider the mnemonic **"COMPLAINS"**:

  Complaint—what is the problem?
  Onset—when did it begin?
  Magnitude—how severe is it?
  Pattern—episodic? crescendo, decrescendo? constant?
  Location—where is it? does it radiate?
  Associated symptoms—are any other symptoms temporally related to the complaint?
  Improvements—what makes it better?
  Negative stimuli—what makes it worse?
  Similar episodes in the past—has it ever happened before?
  Obtaining these descriptive features may reveal the cause of a symptom.
Consider the complaint of chest pain:
  Complaint—chest pain
  Onset—began 2 hours ago
  Magnitude—10/10
  Pattern—crescendo, crushing
  Location—substernal location radiating to the jaw and left arm
  Associated symptoms—shortness of breath, diaphoresis, anxiety
  Improvements—rest, nitroglycerin
  Negative stimuli—exertion
  Similar episodes in the past—5 years ago before coronary artery bypass graft

Chest pain has myriad causes, but the above history strongly points to angina. Consider a different set of features for chest pain:

Complaint—chest pain
Onset—began 6 hours ago
Magnitude—10/10
Pattern—constant, sharp
Location—substernal location, nonradiating
Associated symptoms—inability to take a deep breath
Improvements—sitting-up, leaning forward
Negative stimuli—lying flat
Similar episodes in the past—no prior history

In this instance, the chest pain features are suggestive of pericardial pain, and a different list of diagnostic possibilities should be considered.

Case Discussion

1. Begin with a **summary statement**. After listening to the case, give a one-sentence summary of the case. For example: "The case concerns a 44-year-old male with a history of poorly controlled diabetes and intravenous drug abuse who presents with a 2-day history of fever, rash, and decreasing urine output." The summary statement is a "gestalt," or overall impression, of the case. It is helpful because a presentation often suggests a likely diagnosis, and the discussion can focus on proving or disproving this presumptive diagnosis.

2. Next, make a **problem list** of the major current and past problems. In the above example, a problem list could include:

Fever
Rash
Decreasing urine output
History of diabetes
History of intravenous drug abuse

3. Construct the **differential diagnosis framework** based on the categories of disease or by using mnemonics for specific entities on the problem list.

4. Narrow the diagnostic possibilities based on the history and physical exam.

5. Request specific laboratory or imaging tests to further narrow down the diagnostic possibilities. Specific mnemonics may be used to consider the differential diagnosis for certain laboratory abnormalities. *When new data is not consistent with the diseases being considered, always return to the original, complete differential to reconsider diagnostic possibilities.*

6. Summarize the data and prioritize diagnostic possibilities.

II

PULMONARY AND CRITICAL CARE

General Considerations

General Approach to Pulmonary Disease

Many disorders have pulmonary manifestations, and chest symptoms are frequently the first noticed by the patient (e.g., cough, wheezing, shortness of breath). The lung is a common "target" organ for infection, drug toxicity, cardiovascular compromise, immunologic disease, and neoplastic processes. In approaching the patient with thoracic disease, think of the more common categories of illness, such as infection, neoplasm, toxic exposures, and cardiovascular disease. Also important, but less common, are the immunologic and "exotic" categories of disease, among which there is considerable overlap. Other categories of illness such as endocrine or metabolic diseases have less direct pulmonary involvement. We can apply the mnemonic **"MEDICINE DOC"**:

Metabolic (e.g., amyloidosis, alpha-1-antitrypsin deficiency)
Endocrine (paraneoplastic syndromes, neuroendocrine cell hyperplasia)
Drugs/medicines (e.g., nitrofurantoin, amiodarone, chemotherapy toxicity)
Infection (e.g., HIV-related, TB, bacterial pneumonia)
Congenital (e.g., bronchogenic cysts, Kartagener's, cystic fibrosis)
Immunologic (e.g., Goodpasture's, rheumatoid lung, asthma, BOOP, PIE)
Neoplastic (primary lung, pleural and mediastinal tumors, metastatic disease)
Exotic diseases (e.g., sarcoid, eosinophilic granuloma, LAM, interstitial
    diseases)

Degenerative (e.g., COPD?, degenerative neuromuscular disease [ALS])
Occupational/environmental (e.g., smoking, asbestosis, hypersensitivity)
Cardiovascular (e.g., PE, edema from CHF, VOD, pulmonary hypertension)
Metabolic disorders cause multi-system disease, but the lung and chest usually are not prominently involved. Amyloidosis (also "exotic" and immunologic) may

rarely present as parenchymal or vascular lung disease. Alpha-1-antitrypsin deficiency often leads to emphysema, especially in young smokers, and also could be classified as an inherited disorder. In addition, the lungs may be affected by ongoing metabolic processes, such as pulmonary edema from uremia or tachypnea (Kussmaul breathing) from diabetic ketoacidosis.

The lung has little known **endocrine** function and so this category usually is not helpful in formulating differential diagnoses for chest disease. Lung cancer, particularly small cell carcinoma, can cause paraneoplastic syndromes such as SIADH and Cushing's syndrome. Myxedema may be associated with pleural effusions. The rare entity of neuroendocrine cell hyperplasia may present as chronic obstructive lung disease.

Drugs can cause hypersensitivity reactions. Examples include nitrofurantoin and phenytoin. Also, certain chemotherapeutic agents have well-known pulmonary toxicities (methotrexate, cytoxan, bleomycin, BCNU). Amiodarone causes pulmonary fibrosis as well as other types of lung injury. Intravenous drug abuse and cocaine abuse may have acute and chronic pulmonary manifestations.

Infectious processes of many types can involve the lungs—either primarily, as in lobar bacterial pneumonia, or as part of a disseminated infection, such as aspergillosis in immunocompromised patients. Viruses, mycobacteria, helminths, and other parasites can all cause pulmonary pathology. Certain infectious agents may be specifically associated with chronic diseases, such as PCP in AIDS, or Burkholderia in cystic fibrosis.

The category of **congenital lung disorders** includes anatomic, immunologic, and metabolic abnormalities. Anatomic disorders include bronchogenic cysts, sequestration, and dysmotile cilia syndrome. Immunodeficiency syndromes such as immunoglobulin deficiency or functional neutrophil disorders characteristically present with recurrent sinopulmonary infections. Alpha-1-antitrypsin deficiency predisposes patients to panlobular emphysema. Cystic fibrosis is a common inherited disease with prominent pulmonary involvement including bronchiectasis, chronic infections, and fibrotic changes.

Immunologic disease may affect the lungs specifically, as in asthma, or pulmonary involvement may be only a part of a more widespread immunologic process such as Goodpasture's or Wegener's. Virtually all collagen vascular diseases can involve the respiratory system. Examples include pulmonary fibrosis in scleroderma, lung nodules in rheumatoid arthritis, pleural effusions in SLE, and tracheal collapse in relapsing polychondritis. Neuroimmunologic disorders such as myasthenia gravis and Guillain-Barré may lead to respiratory muscle failure. Tropical eosinophilia represents an immunologic response to the infectious agent filaria, and is treated with the anti-filarial agent diethylcarbamazine. Allergic bronchopulmonary aspergillosis is another example of an infectious agent eliciting an intense inflammatory response. Treatment is primarily directed at modifying the host response with steroids.

Neoplastic disease may arise primarily in the lungs or metastasize from a distant cancer. Neoplasms in other thoracic structures also can affect pulmonary function (e.g., pleural tumors, compression of airways from lymph nodes).

Numerous **exotic conditions** affect the lungs, including histiocytosis X, sarcoidosis, lymphangioleiomyomatosis, and eosinophilic lung disease. Many of these diseases are thought to have an immunologic basis.

Degenerative diseases may cause pulmonary symptomatology secondarily, as is the case with neuromuscular disorders such as ALS. These disorders can lead to swallowing dysfunction and aspiration or respiratory failure. Severe kyphoscoliosis can lead to a restrictive ventilatory defect. Emphysema also could be considered degenerative. In normal aging, lung function slowly declines and is thus degenerative.

In the category of **occupational and environmental exposures**, smoking-related lung disease is very common. Other agents that can cause lung disease are legion and include asbestos, silica, coal dust, and beryllium. Hypersensitivity reactions include farmer's lung, bird-fancier's lung, and numerous other entities. Trauma may lead to hemorrhage, pneumothorax, lung contusion, or injury to other intrathoracic structures.

Cardiovascular diseases may involve the lungs secondarily, causing pulmonary infiltrates and pulmonary hypertension. Abnormalities of the heart and aorta are important considerations in thoracic disease. The vasculitides (classified under immunologic disease) and pulmonary veno-occlusive diseases are more rare. Pulmonary embolism is very common, underdiagnosed, and may be insidious. **The presentations of pulmonary embolism are myriad, and the disorder should be considered in the differential for most thoracic problems.**

General Approach to Critical Care Medicine

The care of critically ill patients is complex and requires an organized approach for managing multi-system disease. Consider the mnemonic "MICU'S LIFE GOALS":

Medications/prophylaxis
Invasions
Cardiovascular
Urine/renal
Skin/decubitis care

Lungs
Infectious disease
Fluids/electrolytes/nutrition
Endocrine

Gastrointestinal/liver
Oncologic/hematologic
Analgesia/neurologic
Long-term prognosis
Social/family

Many of these patients are on numerous **medications** which may cause side effects such as fever, rash, and cytopenias. Carefully review the patient's medicines daily, with an eye toward discontinuing unnecessary agents. Consider all hospitalized patients for some type of DVT prophylaxis, especially ICU patients. Many patients should be considered for stress ulcer/gastritis prophylaxis, as well.

Invasive procedures and in-dwelling lines and catheters are common in the ICU. These **invasions**, while often necessary, are sources of iatrogenic complications, especially infection, and should be discontinued as soon as possible.

A systematic approach is then used to address the patient's problems: **cardiac** (e.g., hemodynamics, diuresis), **urinary/renal** (e.g., fluid balance, BUN/creatinine, dialysis), **skin** (e.g., rash, decubitus care), **lungs** (including ventilator management), **infectious disease** (active or suspected infections, antibiotic therapy including treatment day), **fluids/electrolytes/nutrition** (IVFs, electrolyte disorders or replacement, enteral or parenteral nutrition), **endocrine** (e.g., diabetes, thyroid disease, steroid therapy), **GI/liver** (e.g., gastrointestinal bleeding, diarrhea/constipation, cirrhosis/hepatic dysfunction, pancreatic disease), **oncologic/hematologic** (e.g., malignancies, cytopenias, coagulopathy), and **analgesia/anxiolysis/neurologic status** (e.g., pain management, coma, neurologic deficits, psychiatric disease).

It is important to reassess the **long-term prognosis** frequently so as to avoid futile care. Careful attention often is given to a patient's medical issues without consideration of the likelihood of survival or chance of meaningful recovery. Along the same lines, **social/familial** issues are of paramount importance. Family members often are upset and concerned. They require regular meetings with the ICU physician to discuss medical problems, treatment decisions, prognosis, and end-of-life decisions.

Chest X-Ray Interpretation

Reading a chest x-ray requires an organized approach and can be as easy as **ABCDEF**. . . . Common methods used emphasize starting on the outside and working in or starting in the center and working out. The ABCDEF method* starts with a quick confirmation of the film's qualitative aspects and then outlines a checklist for interpretation.

Initial review:
    AP or PA
    Body position
    Confirm name
    Date
    Exposure
    Films for comparison

---

* This mnemonic was adapted from one proposed by Robert Crauseman, MD.

Interpretation:
   Airway/Adenopathy
   Bones/Breast shadows
   Cardiac silhouette/Costophrenic angles
   Diaphragm/Digestive tract
   Edges/Extra-thoracic tissues
   Fields/Failure

Initially, the reader should look at the film's projection (**AP** or **PA**), then the **body position** (lordotic, rotated, etc.), and then **confirm** the name of the patient, the **date** of the film, and the type of **exposure** (over-penetrated or under-penetrated). See if old **films** are available for a comparison. Again, using ABCDEF as your guide, review the relevant structures on the chest x-ray. Start by looking at the **airway** for width and focal narrowing. Then look for evidence of hilar **adenopathy** or enlargement as might be seen with pulmonary artery hypertension. Next, examine for **breast shadows**, which may affect the density in the lower lung fields, and carefully review the **bones** for rib fractures or evidence of lytic bone lesions.

The **cardiac silhouette** as well as the **costophrenic angles** should be examined for evidence of cardiac enlargement or pleural effusions. Look at the **diaphragm** to see if there is discrepancy in the height of the hemi-diaphragms or evidence of free air under the diaphragm. The **digestive tract** then can be analyzed. Within the chest, look for evidence of esophageal enlargement or herniation of the stomach as well as dilated loops of bowel below the diaphragm. Look at the **edges** and **extra-thoracic tissues**. Particularly, look at the apices for fibrosis or apical disease as well as pneumothoraces, which may occur along the edges apically, laterally, or at the base of the lung. Pleural thickening or plaques may be present. Next, examine the extra-thoracic soft tissues on both the anterior and lateral projections.

Finally, assess the lung **fields** for evidence of alveolar filling or interstitial processes. Evidence of cardiac **failure** may be seen if there is alveolar air space disease with prominent vascularity with or without evidence of pleural effusions.

CHRONIC COUGH

GASPS AND COUGH

Gastroesophageal reflux disease
Asthma
Smoking/chronic bronchitis
Post-infection
Sinusitis/post-nasal drip

Ace-inhibitor
Neoplasm/lower airway lesion
Diverticulum (esophageal)

Congestive heart failure
Outer ear
Upper airway obstruction
GI-airway fistula
Hypersensitivity/allergy

Notes

1. Cough is one of the most common complaints encountered by physicians. It is most often related to upper respiratory tract infections and/or smoking. A persistent cough lasting longer than 2 weeks may indicate a more serious disease. The above differential for chronic cough refers to cases lasting several weeks in which chest radiographs are normal.
2. In a smoker, a chronic cough may indicate chronic bronchitis or it may herald the development of cancer, particularly when it involves an airway. **Any change in the nature of a chronic cough in a smoker warrants investigation for possible neoplasm.**
3. Infections, the most common causes of cough, may be due to viral or bacterial pathogens; viral agents are the usual culprits. In addition, a post-infectious cough may arise due to a cycle of irritation and coughing, which further irritates

the throat. A post-infectious cough may last several weeks after the resolution of the acute infectious process. Treatment consists of cough suppressants, ipratroprium, and, occasionally, a course of inhaled steroids.

4. Both pulmonary parenchymal and pleural disease may present as a cough with or without dyspnea. A chest x-ray usually is the first test obtained after the history and physical in evaluating a chronic cough (i.e., a cough lasting longer than 2 to 3 weeks). If the chest x-ray is negative, consider a more limited differential diagnosis, as outlined by the GASPS AND COUGH mnemonic.

5. Certain historical features may point to the etiology of a chronic cough. Symptoms of heart burn or worsening cough in recumbency (e.g., night) may indicate **gastroesophageal reflux.** A cough that is worse in the evenings or a childhood history of reactive airways disease may suggest **asthma. Smoking-induced** chronic bronchitis and **post-infection** cough from chronic irritation are very common and should be suspected when there is a history of smoking or antecedent infection. Nasal congestion or sensation of post-nasal drip may indicate **sinusitis** as the cause of a cough. Rarely, persistent clear rhinorrhea may be secondary to a CSF leak, which should be considered if nasal drainage and cough don't respond to treatment.

ACE inhibitors, such as captopril, are a common cause of cough in patients on antihypertensive therapy. A **neoplasm** in the lower airway, which is not visible on x-ray, may be made manifest by cough. An esophageal **diverticulum** (e.g., Zenker's diverticulum) causes halitosis, regurgitation, and cough associated with eating. Patients with **congestive heart failure** may have an exacerbation of reactive airways disease with cough and/or wheezing, often worse at night. The presence of ear pain or ear disease should prompt an investigation of the **outer ear** canal and the ear drum, as irritation in those areas by hair, wax, or a foreign body may lead to stimulation of the vagus nerve and cough. The ear canal should be examined in all patients presenting with cough, as ear problems may be asymptomatic.

The presence of stridor on physical examination or a palpable neck mass may indicate an **upper airway** problem as a cause of chronic cough. A **gastrointestinal-airway fistula**, usually tracheoesophageal, characteristically causes cough while eating. And finally, the occurrence of the cough after work or worsening of the cough during the work week may suggest an occupational cause leading to a **hypersensitivity** pneumonitis or an allergy.

6. Studies have shown that patients with cough lasting longer than 3 weeks who come to a pulmonary specialist for evaluation almost invariably have one of four causes of chronic cough: gastroesophageal reflux, asthma, smoking-induced chronic bronchitis, or sinusitis/post-nasal drip. The authors of these studies have suggested that a work-up for these four possible entities and/or empiric treatment of them will lead to resolution of the cough in the great majority of cases. Adding the common entity of post-infectious cough to these four entities creates the mnemonic GASPS, which is a good start for diagnosing the cause of chronic cough.

7. Occasionally, patients with pulmonary fibrosis present with cough and a negative x-ray. These patients usually have fine, "velcro" crackles on chest auscultation, and a CT scan will reveal the interstitial disease.

8. Finally, for patients in whom all other causes of cough are ruled out, a psychogenic etiology is possible. This diagnosis requires exclusion of the other aforementioned etiologies.

CLUBBING

CLUB

Cancer
Liver disease
Ulcerative colitis
Bronchiectasis (especially cystic fibrosis)

Note

Clubbing has been observed in association with lung diseases since antiquity; however, its cause is unknown. It may be seen associated with cancers, particularly pulmonary neoplasms, and when such an association exists, there usually is evidence of hypertrophic pulmonary osteoarthropathy. Clubbing also is observed in some cases of chronic liver disease, as well as in inflammatory bowel disease, especially with ulcerative colitis. Clubbing is a very common symptom in patients with cystic fibrosis and in other patients with bronchiectasis. Other lung diseases that have been associated with clubbing include lung abscess and asbestosis. Less commonly, it has been seen in association with sarcoidosis and eosinophilic granuloma. Clubbing is less commonly associated with pulmonary fibrosis. It is *not* associated with COPD, the presence of clubbing should prompt an investigation for other diagnoses. Clubbing may regress with treatment of the underlying disease.

Dyspnea

SHE PANTS

Stress/anxiety/deconditioning
Heart disease
Emboli

Pulmonary disease
Anemia
Neuromuscular disease
Trachea/upper airway obstruction
Sleep disorder

Notes

1. Dyspnea is defined as an abnormally uncomfortable awareness of breathing and has diverse causes. Patients' own descriptions of symptoms may include fatigue, heavy breathing, weakness, chest tightness, wheezing, and other complaints. There are four primary anatomic areas that influence the sensation of breathing: Pulmonary/airway stretch receptors, Aortic/carotid chemoreceptors, Neuromedullary chemoreceptors and Thoracic muscle stretch receptors ("PANT"). Input from these sites influences the breathing pattern. For example, an acute exacerbation of COPD leads to lung hyperinflation and chest wall expansion, which in turn stimulates pulmonary and thoracic muscle stretch receptors, ultimately leading to the sensation of dyspnea. Neuromuscular disease causes hypoventilation, allowing CO_2 to rise and O_2 to fall. High pCO_2 and low pO_2 stimulate aortic, carotid, and medullary chemoreceptors and cause dyspnea. Alternatively, hypoxia from pulmonary emboli stimulates aortic, carotid, and medullary chemoreceptors and causes dyspnea.

2. The onset of dyspnea (acute, subacute, chronic/progressive) as well as exacerbants should be established. Note that some patients with slowly progressive processes may gradually adapt by decreasing their physical activity, but complain of more acute symptoms at rest. Positional complaints of dyspnea may be elicited, such as **orthopnea** (worsening in the supine position—cardiac disease, upper airway obstruction, diaphragmatic paralysis), **platypnea** (shortness of breath when assuming an upright position—cirrhosis patients with intrapulmonary shunts, pneumonectomy patients with intra-atrial shunts, patients with deficient abdominal musculature), **trepopnea** (dyspnea occurring in the right or left

lateral decubitus position—heart disease, unilateral pulmonary disease), and **paroxysmal nocturnal dyspnea** (most often related to left ventricular failure, but may be seen with obstructive lung disease or sleep-disordered breathing).

3. In addition to exertional and positional precipitants, question the patient about occupational or environmental exposures, animal exposures, inhalational agents, and seasonal worsening.

4. **Stress, anxiety, and deconditioning** are common causes of dyspnea, but often require an extensive investigation to rule out more life-threatening etiologies.

5. Suspect **heart disease** or cardiac ischemia in patients at risk for or with a history of cardiac disease. A history of exertional symptoms, orthopnea, paroxysmal nocturnal dyspnea, or chest pain may be present, as well as physical examination findings of edema, jugulovenous distension, or cardiac murmurs/gallops. Intracardiac shunts also cause hypoxemia, CHF, and dyspnea.

6. Pulmonary **emboli** may present with acute dyspnea, chest pain, or wheezing. Chronic, recurrent pulmonary emboli may be relatively "silent" initially and present as slowly progressive dyspnea. Evidence of lower extremity venous obstruction may not be present.

7. The category of primary **pulmonary disease** includes airway, interstitial and infiltrative, pleural, and pulmonary vascular diseases (embolic disease is considered separately above). Wheezing, cough, and a worsening of symptoms in the evening in a younger person suggest reactive airways disease, while gradually progressive dyspnea and "velcro" crackles in an older patient suggest interstitial pulmonary fibrosis. Primary pulmonary hypertension is often seen in young women and may present as gradually progressive dyspnea with a paucity of physical findings.

8. **Anemia** should be considered in young, menstruating women and in patients with gastrointestinal disease, chronic renal disease, or malignancy.

9. **Neuromuscular diseases** include myopathies, neuropathies, and diaphragmatic dysfunction.

10. Obstruction of the **trachea or upper airways**, may be subtle, and wheezing may be attributed incorrectly to asthma or COPD. Tumors of the upper airway and vocal cord dysfunction are possible etiologies. The flow-volume loop may show a characteristic pattern of obstruction.

11. **Sleep-disordered breathing** is common in obese patients, the elderly, and patients with chronic heart and lung disease. Heavy snoring, jerky limb movements while asleep, morning headaches, daytime hypersomnolence, and sexual dysfunction are clues to the diagnosis. It is important to obtain information from family members and sleep partners as well as the patient. Sleep disturbance can cause fatigue, exercise intolerance, and complaints of dyspnea.

12. One of the most common clinical conundrums is the **differentiation of cardiac from pulmonary dyspnea.** Many patients have both heart and lung disease, and the relative contribution of each may be difficult to discern. The importance of a careful physical examination cannot be overstated. Look carefully for the signs of CHF, including an S3 or S4 gallop, rales, jugulovenous distension (JVD), and peripheral edema. Signs of pulmonary limitation include

wheezing or reduced air entry, increased lung volumes, and hyperresonance to percussion. Note that JVD and pedal edema may be seen with cor pulmonale, and they are not always indicative of left-sided cardiac dysfunction.

In addition to the physical examination, a few simple measurements may be helpful. The peak expiratory flow (PEF) is an easily obtained measure of air flow limitation. A reduction in PEF (< 200 L/min) indicates obstruction and a likely pulmonary etiology. The PaO_2 also tends to be lower in pulmonary dyspnea, although there is considerable overlap. One group of investigators has suggested using a combination of both measures, PEF X PaO_2 / 1000, to differentiate between cardiac and pulmonary dyspnea. They have named this quantity the dyspnea differentiation index (DDI) and use a cut-off of 13 to distinguish between pulmonary and cardiac etiologies. A DDI < 13 indicates a probable pulmonary etiology; values > 13 are suggestive of a cardiac etiology. Be careful to obtain a room air PaO_2 and an accurate PEF (often tachypneic patients cannot perform this test initially) if these parameters are being used.

Another simple bedside parameter is the **blood pressure response to the Valsalva maneuver.** The arterial pressure response to the Valsalva maneuver is abnormal in either systolic or diastolic dysfunction (see Chapter V, Cardiology). Normally, there is a decrease in the pulse amplitude and a narrowing of pulse pressure in response to straining. In CHF this response is blunted, producing a "square wave response." A normal arterial response to Valsalva suggests a pulmonary etiology for dyspnea.

HEMOPTYSIS

CAVITATES

Congestive heart failure
Airway disease/bronchiectasis
Vasculitis/vascular malformations
Infection (e.g., tracheobronchitis, anaerobes, fungi, TB)
Trauma
Anticoagulation
Tumor
Embolism
Stomach (GI or nasal source)

Notes

1. When a patient complains of blood in the sputum, first determine if the source is the lungs or airways (hemoptysis) and not the mouth, nose, pharynx, or GI tract. The next steps are to quantitate the amount of blood and then consider possible etiologies. The disease processes causing hemoptysis often cause tissue necrosis, and the lung **cavitates.** Cavities, cystic changes, bronchiectasis, or alveolar airspace filling on chest x-ray may indicate a source of bleeding. Diffuse infiltrates suggest a more limited differential (e.g., vasculitis with diffuse alveolar hemorrhage, coagulopathy, mitral stenosis). Although an alarming symptom, hemoptysis is often secondary to a benign etiology. Gross or massive hemoptysis is most commonly caused by cancer, TB, or bronchiectasis.

2. **Congestive heart failure** often causes pink, frothy sputum, but rarely frankly bloody sputum. Mitral stenosis is specifically associated with hemoptysis; rarely, mitral regurgitation may cause expectoration of frank blood.

3. Diseases of the **airways** often cause hemoptysis, with tracheobronchitis as the most common cause of blood-tinged sputum. Chronic airway inflammation leads to bronchiectasis, which commonly causes hemoptysis.

4. **Vasculitides**, such as Wegener's granulomatosis or Goodpasture's disease, are often characterized by fever, acute illness, and evidence of systemic involvement, often renal dysfunction. Arteriovenous malformations may cause hemoptysis and should be ruled out before biopsies are taken.

5. Certain **infections**, such as TB, fungi, and anaerobic lung abscess, are more likely to cause hemoptysis. Hemoptysis in these diseases is often seen in association with cystic or cavitary lung disease. Staphylococcal infection following influenza characteristically causes "rusty" or bloody sputum. Rarely, *Serratia marcescens* lung infection causes reddish sputum that appears bloody.

6. **Trauma** from thoracic injuries, inhalations, pulmonary artery catheters, or endotracheal tubes may cause variable amounts of airway bleeding.

7. **Anticoagulation** with coumadin or heparin, or a bleeding diathesis such as thrombocytopenia may precipitate bleeding from the respiratory tract. Again, the presence of blood does not necessarily indicate a malignancy or specific infectious etiology, but be suspicious, since anticoagulation can "unmask" an occult lesion.

8. Suspect **tumors** of the airway or parenchyma in smokers or patients with a known malignancy.

9. Pulmonary **emboli** may cause tissue infarction and hemoptysis. Rarely, pulmonary emboli cause cavitation.

10. Be careful to discriminate hemoptysis from **stomach** or other gastrointestinal bleeding. Nasopharyngeal bleeding may cause cough and be misinterpreted as hemoptysis. The pH of hemoptysis is usually alkaline, while that from the stomach is acidic.

11. The treatment of hemoptysis usually involves observation and perhaps maintaining the bleeding source in the dependent position. If the hemoptysis is

massive (arbitrarily defined as > 500 ml/24 hours), intubation with a double-lumen endotracheal tube is often required, with an attempt to isolate the hemorrhaging lung and prevent "soiling" of the nonbleeding lung. The source of massive bleeding is usually the bronchial arterial system, and hemostasis may be obtained bronchoscopically, surgically, or by invasive radiologic procedure. 12. A more comprehensive list of causes of hemoptysis is outlined below:

TRACHEAL

Tracheobronchitis, **T**rauma, **T**uberculosis, **T**hrombotic thrombocytopenic purpura
Rupture of pulmonary artery (Swan-Ganz), **R**esin/paint production (trimellitic anhydride), **R**asmussen's aneurysm
Aspirated foreign body, **A**llergic bronchopulmonary aspergillosis, **A**naerobic/necrotic pneumonia
Cancer, **C**ardiac (especially mitral stenosis), **C**rack cocaine
Heparin, **H**emosiderosis (idiopathic pulmonary), **H**elminths (paragonimus, echinococcus)
ENT/esophagus (pseudo-hemoptysis), **E**mbolism (pulmonary, septic), **E**ndometriosis
Arteriovenous malformation, **A**rteritis/vasculitis, **A**myloid
Lung abscess, **L**eft atrial myxoma, **L**ithiasis (broncholith), **L**ymphangioleiomyomatosis

Also: penicillamine and arterial bronchial fistula

STRIDOR

WE TRACH OR TREAT

Wegener's
Epiglottitis/supraglottitis

Tracheobronchitis
Relapsing polychrondritis
Aspirated foreign body
Cancer (endotracheal, metastatic, extrinsic compression)
Hereditary (web, Ehlers-Danlos, Williams-Campbell,
  Mounier-Kuhn)

Obstructive lung disease/"dynamic" compression
Reidel's thyroiditis/**R**adiation (fibrosing mediastinitis)

Trauma/**T**racheostomy
Rhinoscleroma
Emotion/anxiety (vocal cord dysfunction)
Amyloidosis
Tracheopathia osteoplastica

WHEEZING

ASTHMA

Asthma
Small airways disease
Tracheal obstruction/large airways disease
Heart failure
Mastocytosis/carcinoid
Anaphylaxis/**A**llergy

Notes

1. "All that wheezes is not asthma" (Osler). The mnemonic ASTHMA emphasizes the *major* causes of wheezing. Wheezing is caused by airway narrowing. The narrowing may be in the upper airway (e.g., laryngeal tumors, vocal cord dysfunction), the large airways (e.g., lung cancer, aspirated foreign body), or the small airways (e.g., bronchiolitis, asthma). When there is upper airway compromise, the wheezing sound is heard best over the trachea and is referred

to as **stridor.** Extra-pulmonary disorders also may cause bronchoconstriction and wheezing. Examples include edema from CHF, anaphylaxis/allergy, and production of bronchoconstricting substances as occurs in the carcinoid syndrome and mastocytosis.

2. **Asthma** is a common cause of wheezing and should be suspected when characteristic history, pulmonary function tests, and response to therapy are seen. When unusual features are encountered, consider other causes of wheezing. Certain asthmatics may be at high risk for respiratory failure and death. A number of factors suggest that asthma is severe and that closer followup and perhaps more intensive therapy and education are necessary:

- Low socioeconomic status
- More than two hospitalizations per year
- A history of intubation
- High number of asthma medications
- Significant diurnal variations of > 30% change per day in airflow
- Nocturnal asthma
- High amount of beta-agonist use (more than two canisters per month)
- Associated psychiatric disease.

Other factors including age, degree of obstruction, and race also can be significant indicators of high-risk asthma.

3. **Small airways diseases** are a group of poorly understood entities distinct from asthma. As the name indicates, they cause narrowing and obstruction of the small airways and consequent wheezing. A relatively common physical examination finding is an end-inspiratory "squeak," which probably corresponds to late opening of distal airways.

4. **Tracheal disease and large airway obstruction** usually cause stridor, which may be difficult to differentiate from wheezing. Upper airway lesions can be detected by physical examination (stridor over the upper airways) or characteristic flow volume loops. A particularly common cause of upper airway wheezing is vocal cord dysfunction. These patients, often young women, typically have exertional or emotionally induced wheezing and shortness of breath which may be severe. Characteristically, the wheezing occurs with inspiration. The flow volume loop may show variability in the inspiratory phase. These patients often are misdiagnosed and treated improperly (often with steroids) as refractory asthmatics. Speech therapy and education are helpful.

5. Extra-pulmonary disorders can cause bronchoconstriction. **Heart failure** may be made manifest by wheezing or it may exacerbate normally quiescent airways hyperreactivity in certain patients. A few unusual diseases (**mastocytosis, carcinoid syndrome**) can produce histaminic compounds that cause rash, hypotension, and wheezing. Carcinoid tumors can cause wheezing by two mechanisms: (1) airway obstruction by a bronchial carcinoid, and (2) production of 5-HIAA, a bronchoconstrictor, which usually only causes wheezing when the tumor involves the liver (see Chapter VI, Endocrinology, the Carcinoid section).

6. **Anaphylaxis and allergy** can cause bronchospasm and wheezing. It is critical to identify environmental precipitants of wheezing, as such knowledge can be life-saving. Avoidance of precipitants obviates the need for medications.

7. Pulmonary function tests are essential in the diagnosis of airway obstruction and assessing the response to therapy. Inspect the flow volume loop with both inspiratory and expiratory limbs for evidence of a large airway obstruction. Obtain lung volume measurements: an obstructive lung disease should show normal or increased lung volumes. Then an assessment of simple spirometry (FEV_1, FVC) determines if obstruction is present. Occasionally, a provocative test for asthma is needed (i.e., methacholine challenge test) when the diagnosis is uncertain.

8. Below is a more comprehensive list of the causes of wheezing:

THE ASTHMATICS

Toxic fumes
Hypersensitivity pneumonitis
Eosinophilic disease

Asthma
Small airways disease
Tracheal obstruction/large airways disease
Heart failure
Mastocytosis/carcinoid
Anaphylaxis/**A**llergy
Thromboembolism
Infection/bronchitis
Cystic fibrosis/bronchiectasis
Smoking/COPD

Acute Respiratory Distress Syndrome— Diffuse Pulmonary Infiltrates

ARDS

Acute onset
Ratio $PaO_2/FiO_2 \leq 200$
Diffuse infiltration
Swan-Ganz wedge < 18 mmHg

Notes

1. The clinical definition of ARDS is: (1) **acute onset**, (2) **ratio (PaO_2/FiO_2)** of 200 or less (regardless of PEEP level), (3) **diffuse, bilateral infiltrates** on frontal chest x-ray, (4) **Swan-Ganz wedge** pressure ≤ 18 mmHg or no clinical evidence of left atrial hypertension.

2. The development of diffuse pulmonary infiltrates may rapidly lead to respiratory failure. Decide whether the etiology is secondary to congestive heart failure or due to capillary leak. Capillary leak leads to the acute respiratory distress syndrome. Diffuse pulmonary infiltrates may be composed of any of the previously mentioned etiologies under pulmonary infiltrate (see previous section).

3. Both congestive heart failure and capillary leak syndromes cause fluid to accumulate in the alveolar space, but the physiologic mechanisms are different. Left heart failure causes an increase in capillary hydrostatic pressure, and fluid is extruded into the alveoli, while ARDS occurs secondary to a capillary leak phenomenon, in which fluid extravasates into the alveoli. The physical examination in a patient in respiratory distress or who is already on a ventilator may be limited, and other diagnostic tests may be needed to indicate the nature of the pulmonary infiltrates.

Two useful tests are the **echocardiogram**, which can give an assessment of overall global cardiac function as well as pulmonary pressures, and **pulmonary** artery catheterization (Swan-Ganz). Although many parameters may be measured with the Swan-Ganz catheter, the most important in differentiating between cardiogenic pulmonary edema and noncardiogenic pulmonary edema are the wedge pressure and pulmonary diastolic pressures. In cardiogenic pulmonary edema, both the wedge and PA diastolic are elevated typically > 20 mmHg. In noncardiogenic pulmonary edema, the pulmonary capillary wedge pressure is usually < 20 mmHg.

4. The therapy of ARDS is supportive, with special emphasis on identifying and treating the cause. There has been a great deal of interest in steroid therapy for ARDS, and current data suggests a role 1–2 weeks after onset, during the so-called fibroproliferative phase. Most studies have shown no salutary effect of steroids when they were started early in the course of ARDS. Further studies are needed to confirm benefit later in the course.

5. Here is a more comprehensive mnemonic for the causes of ARDS:

CARDS? HOPE IT'S NOT ARDS

CNS disorders
Aspiration (especially gastric)
Radiation
Drugs (i.e., heroin, morphine, barbiturates, etc.)
Smoke/toxic gas inhalation

Hypotension/shock
O$_2$ Toxicity
Pancreatitis
Emboli (i.e., pulmonary, fat, amniotic fluid)

Infection/sepsis
Transfusion reaction
Surgery (especially cardiac)

Near drowning
Obstetrical emergencies (e.g., eclampsia, HELLP)
Thermal injury/burns

Altitude sickness
Renal failure
Diffuse intravascular coagulation
Systemic lupus erythematosus

Acute Respiratory Failure

A PE HIT INTUBATED

Aspiration

"White" X-Rays

Pus
Edema

Hemorrhage
Immunologic
Tumor

"Black" X-Rays

Infarcted right ventricle
Neurologic disease (drug overdose, botulism, CVA, Guillain Barré
Tension pneumothorax
Upper airway obstruction (anaphylaxis, foreign body aspiration)
Bronchospasm (COPD exacerbation, asthma)
Arrhythmia
Tamponade
Embolus (pulmonary, air, amniotic fluid, tumor)
Diaphragmatic weakness (surgery/trauma, neurologic disease)

Notes

1. This mnemonic indicates the major causes of acute respiratory failure. The first part of the mnemonic, A PE HIT, indicates the same processes causing pulmonary infiltrates. These processes lead to opacifications on the chest x-ray. The second half of the mnemonic, INTUBATED, indicates etiologies in which the chest x-ray often does not show any infiltrates. In these entities, air space disease is not the cause of respiratory failure, and you must consider other causes of hypoxemia (e.g., neurologic impairment leading to hyperventilation, tension

pneumothorax, upper and lower airway obstruction, and vascular obstruction). Therefore, a common way to divide up the causes of acute respiratory failure is by those that have "white x-rays" (opacifications) and those that have "black x-rays" (clear lung fields).

2. There are six primary mechanisms of hypoxemia:
   - Low inspired fraction of oxygen, such as occurs at high altitude
   - V/Q mismatch
   - Shunt
   - Hypoventilation
   - Diffusion impairment
   - Low mixed venous oxygen.

Of these causes, the most important ones are V/Q mismatch, shunt, and hypoventilation.

3. The indications for emergent endotracheal intubation are:
   - Hypoxemic respiratory failure ($pO_2 < 60$ mmHg on $> 60\%$ oxygen)
   - Hypercarbic respiratory failure (respiratory acidosis with a pH < 7.3)
   - Airway protection
   - Increasing intracranial pressure

BRONCHIECTASIS

A SICK AIRWAY

Airway/lesion/chronic obstruction

Sequestration
Immunodeficiency syndrome (especially immunoglobulin abnormalities)
Cystic fibrosis
Kartagener's syndrome/dysmotile ciliary syndromes

Allergic bronchopulmonary aspergillosis (ABPA)
Infection/**I**nflammation (e.g., tuberculosis, post-viral, whooping cough, collagen-vascular disease)
Reflux (aspiration)/**R**ecurrent injury (heroin, toxic gas inhalation)
Williams-Campbell and other congenital diseases (e.g., Marfan's, Mounier-Kuhn)
Alpha-I antitrypsin deficiency
Yellow nail syndrome, **Y**oung's syndrome

Notes

1. Bronchiectasis, a dilation of the airways, is usually a result of chronic endo-bronchial inflammation.
2. Hemoptysis may be a frequent feature of chronic bronchiectasis.
3. Bronchiectasis leads to dilation of bronchial arteries and increased blood flow, which predisposes patients to bleeding.
4. "Dry" bronchiectasis refers to predominantly upper lobe disease (i.e., secondary to TB or histoplasmosis), which usually drains effectively. The cardinal symptom is hemoptysis. "Wet" bronchiectasis refers to lower lobe disease, which is characterized by chronic cough and purulent sputum. Exceptions to this rough classification include cystic fibrosis, which has prominent upper lobe disease and thick, tenacious secretions.
5. A few diseases commonly cause bronchiectasis with an upper lobe predominance. These can be remembered by the mnemonic **"FACT"** (Fungi, ABPA, Cystic fibrosis, TB)
6. Airway lesions include tumors (benign and malignant), foreign body aspiration, and broncholiths. These airway lesions may cause chronic atelectasis and, ultimately, bronchiectasis.

CAVITARY AND CYSTIC LUNG DISEASE

WEIRD HOLES

Wegener's
Emboli (pulmonary, septic)
Infection (e.g., anaerobes, *Pneumocystis carinii*, TB)
Rheumatoid arthritis (necrobiotic nodules)
Developmental cysts (bronchogenic, sequestration)

Histiocytosis X
Oncologic (primary or metastatic cancer)
Left atrial myxoma (LAM)
Environmental/occupational (silicosis, trauma)
Sarcoidosis

Notes

1. The presence of cavities or cystic changes on the chest x-ray may be caused by necrotizing processes such as infections, vasculitides, infarction from emboli, or malignancy. Also consider certain developmental anomalies, occupational exposures, and unusual primary lung diseases.

2. Pulmonary cavities primarily result from six sections of the "MEDICINE DOC" mnemonic: (1) Infectious, (2) Congenital, (3) Immunologic, (4) Neoplastic, (5) Exotic, (6) Occupational/environmental exposures.

3. **Infectious etiologies** include mycobacterial disease, fungal disease, necrotizing bacterial infections, parasitic infections, and septic pulmonary emboli. Tuberculous cavities typically occur in the upper lobes, but can present in any location. They are part of a chronic disease process, so prior films are helpful in analyzing the progression of the disease. In the absence of superinfection, air-fluid levels are uncommon in tuberculous cavities. Sputum analysis often is positive in active cavitary tuberculosis, as the organism load is relatively high within the cavity. Fungal diseases, such as coccidiomycosis, blastomycosis, and histoplasmosis, also can produce cavities

Aspergillosis may cause an acute necrotizing pneumonia in immunocompromised patients, or it may colonize pre-existing cavities, producing a visible fungal ball on chest radiography. Because invasive aspergillosis characteristically involves blood vessels, thrombosis, infarction, and cavity formation often ensue. The characteristic "crescent" sign is produced by infarcted tissue within the fungal cavity.

Virtually all bacterial infections can cause a pneumonia that may produce cavitary lung changes. Cavitary changes are more typical of anaerobes and gram-negative organisms. However, *Staphylococcus aureus*, *Streptococcus pneumonia*, and Legionella species all can produce cavitary lung changes. A rare complication of bacterial pneumonia is pulmonary gangrene. The radiologic appearance can be characteristic, with infarcted lung tissue floating within a parenchymal cavity. Surgery often is required for resolution.

Parasitic infections should be suspected in individuals with appropriate travel and exposure history. Paragonimiasis is secondary to a liver fluke and is endemic to Southeast Asia. Echinococcus is associated with exposure to sheep, dogs, or wild hosts such as caribou or reindeer. A characteristic radiologic appearance, the "water-lily" sign, is produced when the encysted organisms' membranes detach from the adventitia and float within a cavity.

Finally, septic pulmonary emboli most commonly occur as a result of tricuspid endocarditis or a peripheral source. Multiple cavitary lesions may be present, often in the lower lung zones where the blood supply is greater.

4. Congenital anomalies include **developmental cysts** (e.g., bronchogenic) as well as pulmonary sequestration, and should be suspected in young adults presenting with asymptomatic cavitary lung lesions.

5. Immunologic processes include the vasculidities and rheumatoid arthritis. **Wegener's granulomatosis** is the most common immunologic disease that presents

with pulmonary cavities. **Rheumatoid arthritis** can cause lung nodules that feature central necrosis and eventually cavitate. Ankylosing spondylitis and polymyositis also may feature apical bullous disease.

6. Oncologic processes can produce cavities by two mechanisms: (1) obstruction of a bronchus with distal suppurative infection, or (2) cavitation of the tumor mass secondary to outgrowing of the blood supply. Squamous cell carcinomas have a particular propensity to outgrow their blood supply and cavitate. Angiocentric lymphoma (lymphomatoid granulomatosis) is an unusual malignancy that can cause multiple lung masses which may cavitate.

7. Exotic diseases causing cysts include **histiocytosis X, LAM,** and **sarcoidosis.** Younger patients who present with multiple lung cysts should be suspected of having these diseases. Histiocytosis X, also called eosinophilic granuloma, is a disease of smokers. LAM is related to tuberous sclerosis and occurs in young females.

8. Environmental or occupational exposures may lead to cystic lung disease. A common occupational cause of cystic lung disease is silicosis, which occurs in hard rock miners. Also, rarely, multiple trauma patients develop acute cavitary lung disease of uncertain etiology. Presumably, the trauma leads to vascular injury, resulting in the cavitary changes on x-ray.

9. As with most respiratory problems, **emboli** are a possible, albeit rare, cause of cystic or cavitary changes. Both pulmonary and septic emboli can cause necrosis, infarction, and subsequent cavitation.

INTERSTITIAL LUNG DISEASE

IS IT IPF?

IPF
Sarcoidosis

Inhalational (pneumoconioses)
Treatment-related (e.g., medications, radiation, chemotherapy)

Immunologic (collagen-vascular diseases)
Post-inflammatory (e.g., infection, ARDS)
Familial

Notes

1. The lung interstitium is the area between the gas-exchanging alveolar epithelium and the capillary membrane. Normally this space is very thin and allows for effective gas exchange. When diseases or toxins damage the interstitium, it may become infiltrated with inflammatory cells and, ultimately, scar tissue. These interstitial lung diseases produce an impairment in the diffusion of oxygen and lead to respiratory symptomatology. The chest radiograph characteristically shows what is often called a reticular or linear pattern of infiltration.

The term "diffuse parenchymal lung disease" may be more appropriate since these diseases may involve the airways and airspaces in addition to the interstitium. The mnemonic "IS IT IPF?" summarizes the primary causes of interstitial disease.

2. One of the most commonly encountered interstitial lung diseases is idiopathic pulmonary fibrosis, **IPF**. **Sarcoidosis** is also very common and has myriad systemic manifestations. **Immunologic/collagen-vascular diseases** have well-described systemic features and pulmonary involvement. Lung disease is occasionally the initial finding in patients with collagen-vascular diseases. **Treatment-related** causes must be carefully considered since removal of the offending agent is critical. A complete occupational and environmental history is mandatory to exclude **inhalational lung disease**. Avoidance of the inciting agent is mandatory for the patient, and other persons at risk may be identified. Pulmonary infections, ARDS, and other lung injuries may result in **post-inflammatory** fibrosis and permanent parenchymal changes. Finally, a number of unusual **familial** diseases have associated interstitial lung disease.

3. The history and clinical examination sometimes suggest an etiology for interstitial disease, such as an exposure or an underlying disease. The chest radiograph may show characteristic patterns which may also suggest an etiology. For example, certain diseases more commonly have predominantly **upper lobe** involvement, including Ankylosing spondylitis, PIE (chronic eosinophilic pneumonia), Infections (TB, histoplasmosis), Coal worker's pneumoconiosis/silicosis, Eosinophilic granuloma (histiocytosis X), and Sarcoidosis/berylliosis ("**APICES**"). A predominantly **lower lobe** pattern of disease is seen in asbestosis, alveolar proteinosis, IPF, collagen-vascular diseases, and chronic hypersensitivity pneumonitis. Nodules suggest sarcoidosis, Wegener's, inhalational exposures (pneumoconioses), rheumatoid arthritis, or lymphomatoid granulomatosis ("**SWIRL**"). The presence of **pleural disease** is unusual in interstitial lung disease, but may be seen in asbestosis, lymphangitic carcinomatosis, and collagen vascular diseases. Normal or increased lung volumes and cystic changes are seen in only a few diseases. Finally, **lymphadenopathy** is also unusual in interstitial lung disease and may indicate sarcoidosis, amyloidosis, lymphangitic carcinomatosis, or berylliosis.

4. Diffuse parenchymal lung disease most often leads to increased lung elasticity and a reduction in lung volumes. Pulmonary function tests usually reveal a restrictive ventilatory defect. Occasionally interstitial disease is seen in a patient

with **normal or increased lung volumes**, and this narrows the differential considerably. The causes of interstitial lung disease with normal or increased lung volumes are summarized by the mnemonic **LET'S BRONCH:** LAM, Eosinophilic granuloma (histiocytosis X), Talc injection (intravenous drug abuse), Sarcoidosis, Bronchiectatic diseases (e.g., cystic fibrosis), Respiratory bronchiolitis, Obliterative bronchiolitis, Neurofibromatosis, COPD + ILD, Hypersensitivity pneumonitis. (This mnemonic is adapted from one invented by Robert Shpiner, MD.) In contrast to other causes of interstitial lung disease, these diseases feature obstruction on pulmonary function tests. Exceptions are hypersensitivity pneumonitis and eosinophilic granuloma, which most often show restriction on pulmonary function testing despite normal or increased lung volumes.

5. There are approximately 180 known individual diseases that may be associated with interstitial lung disease. The most frequently encountered are IPF, sarcoidosis, and interstitial lung disease associated with collagen vascular diseases. The following mnemonic lists many of the causes of interstitial lung disease:

I HAVE BRONCHED AN INTERSTITIAL LUNG

Idiopathic pulmonary fibrosis (IPF)

Hermansky-Pudlak syndrome
ARDS recovery
Veno-occlusive disease
End-stage liver disease

Bronchocentric granulomatosis
Rheumatoid arthritis and other collagen vascular diseases
Organic and inorganic dusts (occupational/ environmental)
Niemann-Pick and Gaucher's diseases
Congestive heart failure
Hypereosinophilic syndrome
Eosinophilic lung diseases (PIE syndromes)
Drug exposures (e.g., amiodarone, gold, antibiotics, chemotherapy)

Amyloidosis
Neoplastic (lymphangitic carcinomatosis, post-radiation therapy)

Idiopathic pulmonary hemosiderosis
Neurofibromatosis
Tuberous sclerosis
Eosinophilic granuloma/histiocytosis X
Renal failure/uremia
Sarcoidosis
Transplantation (GVHD)
Infections (residua of active infection of any type)
Toxic chemicals (gases, fumes, vapors, aerosols,
    paraquat, radiation)
Idiopathic hypereosinophilic syndrome
Alveolar proteinosis
Lymphangioleiomyomatosis (LAM)

Lymphocytic disorders (e.g., pseudolymphoma,
    lymphocytic interstitial pneumonitis)
Ulcerative colitis and other gastrointestinal diseases
Necrotizing vasculitis (Wegener's, Churg-Strauss,
    lymphomatoid granulomatosis)
Goodpasture's disease and other pulmonary
    hemorrhage syndromes

MEDIASTINAL MASS

CHEST ALARMS

Cysts (bronchial, pericardial)
Hernias (Bochdalek, Morgagni)
Esophageal diverticulum
Schwannoma/neurogenic tumors
Ts (The 4 T's: teratoma, thymona, thyroid, and terrible
    lymphoma)

Aneurysms (aortic and pulmonary)
Lymph node enlargement
Adipose tissue
Renal (intrathoracic kidney)
Metastatic disease
Splenosis/extramedullary hematopoesis

Notes

1. One of the most common disorders of the mediastinum is a mass. The first step in evaluation is to determine the compartment of the mediastinum in which the mass is located: anterior, middle, or posterior. The most common **anterior masses** are the 4 Ts: thymona, thyroid mass, teratoma, terrible lymphoma. The most common **middle masses** are vascular masses, lymph node enlargements, or cysts (pericardial, bronchogenic). **Posterior masses** include neurogenic tumors, hiatal hernias, or esophageal diverticuli.
2. A CT scan, followed by biopsy when appropriate, is the usual approach to diagnosis.
3. Causes of a mediastinal mass, by compartment, are summarized by the mnemonic below. There is some overlap in the categories as some entities can be found in more than one mediastinal compartment.

NERVES AND CHEST PARTS

Posterior Mediastinum
Neurogenic tumors
Esophageal enlargement or diverticulum
Renal (intrathoracic kidney)
Vascular (e.g., descending aortic aneurysm)
Extramedullary hematopoesis/splenosis
Skeletal/spinal (e.g., vertebral osteophyte, meningocele)

Middle Mediastinum
Adipose tissue ("fat pad")
Nodes
Dilated aortic root

Cysts (pericardial, bronchogenic)
Hematoma (e.g., after surgery or line placement)
Enlarged pulmonary arteries
Stomach (hiatal hernia)
Tumor (metastatic, primary)

Anterior Mediastinum

Parathyroid mass
Aortic arch aneurysm
Right ventricular enlargement
Ts (teratoma, thymona, thyroid, terrible lymphoma)
Subclavian catheter hematoma

PLEURAL EFFUSION

PE HIT? DECUB, TAP

Pus
Edema

Hemorrhage
Immunologic
Tumor

Dialysis (peritoneal)
Esophagus (Boerhaave's)
Chyle
Urine
Bile

Total parenteral nutrition
Ascites
Pancreatic

Notes

1. There are many different types of fluid that may enter the pleural space. Similar to pulmonary infiltrates, pleural fluid may consist of **pus, edema, hemorrhage, immunologic reactions**, or **tumor cells** (PE HIT). These are the major causes of fluid in the pleural space. However, other types also may gain access, such as **dialysis fluid**, inflammatory fluid from a ruptured **esophagus, chyle** from injury to the thoracic duct, **urine, bile, total parenteral nutrition (TPN), ascitic fluid**, or **pancreatic fluid** (DECUB TAP). There even have been cases of CSF (pleuro-duro fistula) and stool (fecothorax) in the pleural space. As with pulmonary infiltrates, pulmonary embolism must be considered in the differential diagnosis of a pleural effusion.

2. When a pleural effusion is discovered, decubitus films should be obtained to see if the fluid flows freely. Thoracentesis should then be performed *without delay* on freely flowing fluid. Thoracentesis is indicated in virtually all newly diagnosed, free-flowing pleural effusions. Exceptions to this rule are when the clinical diagnosis is certain (e.g., CHF) or there is only a small amount of fluid in the pleural space.

3. Pleural effusions are broadly categorized as transudates or exudates. Transudates occur when **systemic factors** that influence the formation and absorption of pleural fluid are altered. The most common causes are left ventricular failure, pulmonary embolus, and cirrhosis. Others include nephrotic syndrome, peritoneal dialysis, myxedema, atelectasis, and urinothorax. Urinothorax is the only cause of an acidic transudate.

4. Exudates occur when **local factors** that influence the formation and absorption of pleural fluids are altered. The most common causes are bacterial pneumonia, malignancy, viral infection, and pulmonary embolus. Pulmonary embolus may cause either a transudate or an exudate depending on whether infarction and hemorrhage occurs. Cancer and hypothyroidism also may cause either a transudate or exudate.

5. Criteria for an exudate are:
   a. Pleural fluid protein/serum protein > 0.5
   b. Pleural fluid LDH/serum LDH > 0.6
   c. Pleural fluid LDH > 2/3 of the normal upper limit for serum.
Transudates have none of these features.

6. If the fluid is exudative, the following tests should be ordered: glucose, amylase, cell count and differential, cultures, cytology, gram stain, and pH. Two or three cytologic samples will rule out a malignancy in most cases.

7. A possible parapneumonic effusion should be tapped immediately. It is said to be "complicated" if any of the following are present:
   a. Gross pus
   b. Organisms visible on gram stain
   c. Glucose < 50
   d. pH < 7.0
Complicated effusions usually require chest tube drainage.

8. TB pleuritis usually requires a pleural biopsy for diagnosis due to the scarcity of organisms in the fluid. The fluid often (but not always) lacks mesothelial cells. Making the diagnosis of primary tuberculous pleuritis may be difficult, but it should be pursued aggressively as there is a high incidence of progression to pulmonary parenchymal disease. The diagnosis may be elusive: several new diagnostic studies are available. There is evidence that an elevated adenosine deaminase level may be helpful in establishing a diagnosis of tuberculous pleuritis. A second promising diagnostic test is a polymerase chain reaction assay specific for mycobacterial disease. This test may be applied to sputum samples and has been used for analysis of pleural and other body fluids. It has a high degree of sensitivity, with probably a lesser degree of specificity.

9. A low glucose is characteristic of rheumatoid arthritis effusions. Other entities that may have a very low glucose include empyema, malignancy, tuberculosis, SLE, and esophageal rupture.

10. Bloody fluid may be seen in many conditions, but an RBC count greater than 100,000 suggests trauma, malignancy, pulmonary embolism, post cardiac injury syndrome, or asbestos pleuritis (**IT BLED**—Intravenous catheter, Trauma, BAPE [benign asbestos pleural effusion], Lung cancer, Embolism, Dressler's syndrome).

11. A pleural fluid amylase level occasionally is helpful. The mnemonic **AMYLASE UP** (Adenocarcinoma, Mycobacteria, Yorking (esophageal rupture), Liver disease, Acute pancreatitis, Serum hyperamylasemia, Ectopic pregnancy, Ureteral obstruction, Pseudocyst) can help you remember related disorders. Hydronephrosis and other disease states that lead to an elevated serum amylase also increase the pleural fluid amylase level. The highest levels are seen in pancreatic disease, and usually are greater than 20. In other causes including cancer the pleural fluid/serum amylase level is usually about 10. Pancreatic pseudocysts typically have the highest amylase levels, often greater than 100,000. Amylase isozyme analysis may be helpful in pinpointing the cause of a high pleural fluid amylase. A high salivary isozyme level indicates malignancy, whereas a high pancreatic isozyme level indicates pancreatic disease. The most common malignancies causing a high pleural fluid amylase are lung or ovarian carcinoma. This fact can be helpful in differentiating lung carcinoma from mesothelioma, because mesotheliomas do not make amylase.

12. A high percentage of eosinophils in the pleural space usually indicates the presence of air or blood. Eosinophils may accumulate after a pneumothorax or hemorrhage into the pleural space. Other causes of pleural fluid eosinophilia include certain drugs such as dantrolene, pulmonary emboli, parasitic infections, fungal infections, and malignancies. Benign asbestos pleural effusion (BAPE) is a complication of asbestos exposure that may occur 10–15 years after the initial exposure. Because the pleural effusion is bloody, a high eosinophil count may be seen with BAPE as well. The mnemonic **BAPE** (Blood, Air, Parasites, Emboli) summarizes the primary causes of pleural fluid eosinophilia.

13. Suspect the presence of lymphatic fluid in the pleural space (chylothorax) when effusions re-accumulate rapidly or have a milky color. The fluid is not always milky, however, and may be turbid or bloody. Conditions that commonly lead to the accumulation of lymphatic fluid (chyle) include trauma, malignancy (especially lymphoma), chest surgery, coughing, vomiting, or straining. A great number of other conditions may be associated with a chylothorax as well, including LAM; yellow nail syndrome; infections leading to thoracic lymphadenopathy, including tuberculosis and fungal infections; filariasis; aortic and pulmonary aneurysms; and certain congenital syndromes, for example Down's syndrome, Noonan's syndrome, and Turner's syndrome.

Some major etiologies of chylothorax are summarized by the mnemonic CHYLES—Cough/strain/vomiting, Hereditary diseases, Yellow nail syndrome, Lymphoma/LAM/lymph node enlargement, Elephantiasis, Surgery/trauma. All of these conditions lead to obstruction of lymphatics and/or injury to the thoracic duct. A pleural fluid triglyceride level > 110 establishes the diagnosis of chylothorax. A level at 50–110 is intermediate and may be indicative of chylothorax. When the level is intermediate, the pleural fluid should be submitted for electrophoresis to look for the presence of chylomicrons. When a chylothorax is diagnosed, establish NPO for the patient, and initiate TPN. Do not attempt aggressive chest tube drainage, as this may lead to nutritional depletion. The thoracic duct may then spontaneously heal; if it does not, surgical ligation may be indicated.
14. If the cause of a pleural effusion is not determined after thoracentesis, then pleural biopsy is usually the next diagnostic step. If pleural biopsy fails to yield a diagnosis, then consider an open surgical procedure. Bronchoscopy may be helpful if there is another confirmed pulmonary lesion or hemoptysis, but the yield is quite low for an undiagnosed pleural effusion with an otherwise normal x-ray.
15. A small number of exudative effusions elude diagnosis even after open pleural biopsy. Experience shows that about two-thirds of these do not recur, and no diagnosis is established. They are presumed to be a result of infection or other inflammatory process that has resolved. The remaining one-third of cases are eventually found to have a specific diagnosis. Malignancy, usually lymphoma, is the most common cause. A few patients eventually are diagnosed with collagen vascular diseases or other miscellaneous diagnoses. Interestingly, in the largest published series, none of the patients with undiagnosed exudative pleural effusions who had surgical biopsy were ever found to have tuberculosis.
16. Here is a longer list of the causes of pleural effusions:

UH, DOC I'LL NEED MY TAP STAT

Urinothorax
Hypothyroidism

Drugs (e.g., nitrofurantoin, amiodarone, procarbazine, dantrolene, methylsergide)
Ovarian hyperstimulation syndrome
Collagen vascular disease

Infection (pneumonia, parapneumonic effusion, emphysema, TB)
Left ventricular failure
Lymphangioleiomyomatosis

Nephrotic syndrome
Esophageal rupture
Embolism (PE)
Dialysis (peritoneal)

Malignancy (primary, metastatic, Meig's syndrome)
Yellow nail syndrome

Trauma (hemothorax)
Ascites (hepatic or pancreatic)
Post-surgical

SVC obstruction (or other great veins)
Trapped lung
Asbestos (BAPE)
TPN

PNEUMOTHORAX

CHEST PAINS

Cystic lung disease (e.g., cystic fibrosis, LAM, histiocytosis X, bullous emphysema)
Hereditary connective tissue diseases (Marfan's, Ehlers-Danlos, pseudoxanthoma elasticum)
Endometriosis (catamenial)
Spontaneous
Trauma

Pneumonia, **P**CP
Altitude, **A**lveolar microlithiasis
Iatrogenic (thoracentesis, central line, ventilator, postoperative)
Neoplasm (rare—osteogenic carcinoma metastases)
Scleroderma, **S**arcoidosis

Notes

1. Primary or "spontaneous" pneumothorax commonly occurs in tall, thin individuals and is usually due to rupture of apical blebs. Smokers are at increased risk.
2. Treatment of a large pneumothorax initially involves aspiration, often followed by chest tube re-expansion. Recurrent pneumothorax can be treated with sclerosing agents (tetracycline or bleomycin) or surgically. A small pneumothorax can be followed by serial chest x-rays, because it may resolve without medications or treatment.
3. Tension pneumothorax is life threatening and can lead to cardiac arrest. It may be a complication of mechanical ventilation. It is treated emergently with a large-bore needle placed in the pleural space.

PULMONARY HYPERTENSION

LVEDP

Left-sided failure
Vascular disease/obstruction
Extrinsic compression
Desaturation/hypoxia
Pulmonary parenchymal disease

PA HTNS

Pulmonary parenchymal disease/primary pulmonary
   hypertension
Apnea/**A**noxia

Heart failure
Thromboembolism
Neuromuscular/skeletal disease
Scleroderma/vasculitis

Notes

1. The differential diagnosis for pulmonary hypertension (PA HTNS) is a "plumb-ing" problem. The history, physical examination, and chest x-ray guide you in determining where the "block" in the plumbing is located (i.e., aorta, aortic valve, left ventricle, mitral valve, left atrium, large pulmonary veins, pulmonary venules, pulmonary capillaries, pulmonary arterioles, pulmonary arteries). Also consider pulmonary valve disease, right ventricular dysfunction, tricuspid valve disease, right atrial disease, and subclavian vein thrombosis.

2. Left ventricular failure is the most common cause of pulmonary hypertension. In left-sided failure, the left ventricular end-diastolic pressure (LVEDP) is elevated. Thus, an important first step is to assess left ventricular function to rule-out a cardiac cause of pulmonary hypertension. The physical examination may detect an S_4 or pulmonary edema, suggesting left ventricular failure. Physical findings indicative of pulmonary hypertension of any cause include jugulovenous distension, a right ventricular heave, a loud P_2, and a systolic pulmonary murmur.

3. Causes of **left-sided failure** (post-pulmonary capillary) include systolic and diastolic CHF, congenital heart disease, valvular heart disease, and atrial tumors. **Vascular causes** of pulmonary hypertension include chronic thromboemboli, primary pulmonary hypertension, intravenous drug abuse, collagen-vascular diseases such as scleroderma/CREST, schistosomiasis, diet/weight-loss pills, sickle cell anemia, and pulmonary hypertension associated with cirrhosis. Pulmonary venous disease is rare and, although vascular, it is a post-pulmonary capillary process that may look like CHF. **Extrinsic processes** causing pulmonary hypertension include kyphoscoliosis, neuromuscular disease, and fibrosing mediastinitis. Periodic oxygen **desaturation** caused by obstructive sleep apnea or hypoventilation syndromes eventually cause pulmonary hypertension. Chronic hypoxia of any cause leads to pulmonary vascular constriction and, ultimately, hypertension. Finally, **pulmonary parenchymal diseases** such as COPD and interstitial lung disease destroy the capillary bed, leading to pulmonary hypertension.

4. An echocardiogram demonstrates both LV and RV function, valvular function, and an estimate of pulmonary artery pressures; it is a good initial noninvasive test. Definitive localization of the "block" may require pulmonary artery catheterization to measure the pulmonary capillary wedge pressure (PCWP), a reflection of left atrial pressure, and an indicator of LVEDP. Pulmonary angiography may be necessary to rule out chronic pulmonary emboli or other vascular obstructions. The mnemonic below lists the causes of pulmonary hypertension and indicates the helpful diagnostic information provided by the PA catheter.

I CHECK PCWPS AND LVEDPS

Interstitial lung disease

Chronic obstructive pulmonary disease
Hyperthyroidism
Emboli (chronic pulmonary emboli, intravenous drug
    abuse)
Collagen-vascular diseases
Kyphoscoliosis

Primary pulmonary hypertension (including pulmonary
    capillary hemangiomatosis)
Congenital heart disease
Worms (e.g., schistosomiasis)
Pulmonary veno-occlusive disease
Sleep apnea

Atrial disease
Neuromuscular disease
Diet pills (aminorex)

Liver disease/cirrhosis
Valvular heart disease
Extrinsic compression of pulmonary vasculature
    (e.g., fibrosing mediastinitis)
Diastolic inhibition/equalization (tamponade,
    constrictive pericarditis)
Primary cardiomyopathy (dilated, restrictive, infiltrative)
Sickle cell anemia

Pulmonary Infiltrate

A PE HIT?

Aspiration

Pus
Edema

Hemorrhage
Immunologic
Tumor

Notes

1. A pulmonary infiltrate is a common medical problem. Although the potential etiologies are many, the composition of infiltrates is limited. A pulmonary infiltrate may be composed of: (1) **aspirated** food or oil, (2) **pus** (infection), (3) pulmonary **edema** or vascular leak, (4) **hemorrhage**, (5) certain **immunologic** processes including collagen vascular diseases, eosinophilic lung diseases, BOOP, and alveolar proteinosis, and (6) **tumor** infiltration. As the mnemonic suggests, always consider **pulmonary embolism** in the differential diagnosis of a new infiltrate, particularly when risk factors are present or the clinical picture is unclear.

2. A patient's specific presenting symptoms can indicate the nature of the infiltrate. For example, fever and productive cough may indicate an infectious etiology. On the other hand, a patient with rales and a history of congestive heart failure most likely has pulmonary edema. Hemoptysis may indicate an underlying pulmonary hemorrhage syndrome, while the presence of certain systemic symptoms may point toward an immunologic cause of the lung disease. Finally, risk of lung cancer or characteristic radiographs may lead to a consideration of neoplasm. Pulmonary neoplasms often block an airway, leading to a post-obstructive pneumonia, which may be recurrent or fail to clear after appropriate therapy. Less commonly, neoplasms primarily involve the airspaces and cause an infiltrate (see below). Neoplasms can have the same effect by bleeding into the airspaces.

3. Community-acquired, bacterial pneumonia (CAP) is the most common cause of a pulmonary infiltrate. The typical presenting features are fever, cough with purulent sputum, and a lobar infiltrate. Multi-lobar disease is more serious and less common. With timely and effective antimicrobial therapy, clinical and radiographic improvement are evident. Of course, there are exceptions to these rules depending on host-specific factors (e.g., the elderly) and the particular pathogen (e.g., Legionella), but they provide valuable guidelines in assessing response.

4. A common clinical problem is differentiating between CAP and other causes of air-space disease. When faced with a pulmonary infiltrate, there are four primary considerations: **C**linical presentation, **U**nderlying diseases/risks, **R**adiographic appearance, and **E**xpected response to therapy (**CURE**). The **clinical presentation** of CAP usually includes acute onset of fever, cough, and purulent sputum. The absence of these features or the presence of less typical findings (e.g., prolonged course, hemoptysis, lymphadenopathy, disproportionate hypoxemia) should prompt consideration of other entities. A particular patient's **underlying diseases or risk factors** (e.g., AIDS, known malignancy, smoking/COPD, immobility/hypercoagulability, medications/drug use) predispose to specific pathogens or conditions other than CAP. The **radiographic pattern** of the infiltrate may suggest a specific diagnosis (e.g., volume loss, peripheral pattern, recurrence in the same area). And, finally, has the patient had the **expected response to therapy**, or has the infiltrate persisted or increased in size?

An algorithm based on these principal considerations begins with empiric therapy for CAP when the radiograph and symptoms are reasonably suggestive. If the patient responds to treatment and radiographic clearing occurs, then no further investigation is needed. If atypical features are present, progression or recurrence occurs, or there is no improvement, then consider other etiologies.

5. When a pulmonary infiltrate progresses or fails to resolve after specific therapies, consider the causes of chronic pulmonary infiltrates summarized by the mnemonic **ALVEOLAR LIST**: **A**lveolar cell carcinoma, **L**ymphoma, **V**asculitis, **E**osinophilic pneumonia, **O**rganizing pneumonia, **L**ipoid pneumonia, **A**lveolar proteinosis, **R**eflux/aspiration, **L**IP/DIP (lymphocytic and desquamative interstitial pneumonitis), **I**nfection (e.g., TB, fungi), **S**arcoidosis, and **T**racheobronchial obstruction. This mnemonic refers to the fact that the majority of these entities show an **alveolar-filling pattern** on chest x-rays. A few other etiologies may rarely cause a chronic alveolar infiltrate, including amyloidosis, alveolar microlithiasis, and silent mitral stenosis.

6. The following mnemonic offers a more detailed summary of the causes of pulmonary infiltrates:

CAN IT BE A PE?

CHF (pulmonary edema)
Aspiration (e.g., food, oil , GERD)
Neoplasm (airway obstruction, bronchoalveolar cell carcinoma, lymphoproliferative disorders)

Infection (bacterial, fungal, viral, mycobacterial, protozoal, helminthic)
T-cells/B-cells (LIP, sarcoidosis, hypersensitivity pneumonitis)

BOOP (organizing pneumonia)
Eosinophils (PIE syndromes)

Alveolar hemorrhage (e.g., vasculitis, coagulopathy, focal processes)

Protein (alveolar proteinosis)
Embolus (e.g., thromboemboli, tumor emboli, septic emboli)

PULMONARY NODULE

A NODULE

Age

Nicotine
Old Films
Doubling time
Underlying diseases
Lymph nodes
Examinations

Notes

1. The finding of a solitary pulmonary nodule is cause for concern. The potential etiologies are many, and some major causes are summarized in note number 11. Even this long list is not comprehensive, and so a more practical approach to the solitary pulmonary nodule is outlined by the mnemonic A NODULE.
2. The most critical questions to answer are whether or not the nodule represents a malignancy and if surgery is indicated. Several historical elements increase the chance of a malignancy, and a stepwise approach also is outlined by the mnemonic above.
3. An **age** greater than 35 increases the chance of malignancy. Therefore, a more aggressive diagnostic strategy may be undertaken in an older patient.
4. **Nicotine** addicts (smokers) have a greatly increased incidence of bronchogenic carcinoma. A smoking history mandates a more aggressive approach.

5. One of the first things to find out is whether or not **old films** are available, to determine if the nodule is a new finding. A lesion that was present on an old film is much less likely to be malignant.

6. The **doubling time** of a nodule may indicate whether or not it is likely to be malignant. Malignancies usually double in size after 20 days but before 450 days. Benign lesions may greatly increase in size in less than 20 days and often are due to infections. Also, any lesion that does not double in 450 days is much less likely to be malignant.

7. Consider the patient's **underlying diseases**. Is this patient a smoker with emphysema and at increased risk for cancer? Does the patient have a known malignancy? Evidence of pneumonia and infection? Evidence of a collagen vascular disease or an immunodeficiency syndrome? Many historical features are indicative of specific etiology for the nodule.

8. Physical examination may reveal **lymphadenopathy** indicative of malignancy or infection. Also, if a lymph node is detected, this should be the first site of biopsy. It will be easier to biopsy than the lung lesion and will establish staging.

9. Finally, diagnostic **examinations** should be undertaken. The choice of tests depends, of course, on the patient and the above-mentioned risk factors, which will determine how aggressive the physician can be in trying to identify whether or not the lesion is malignant. Examinations include CT scans, fine needle aspiration of the lesion, bronchoscopy with biopsy, thoracotomy with biopsy, or, in some cases, mediastinoscopy. Recent evidence has shown that PET scanning may be able to differentiate malignant from benign lesions.

10. The finding of multiple nodules indicates different types of disease. The categories of disease to be considered include developmental abnormalities, infectious diseases, immunologic diseases, metastatic neoplasms, and traumatic injury, as well as idiopathic causes. In AIDS patients, multiple nodules may occur secondary to PCP, tuberculosis, cryptococosis, CMV, Kaposi's sarcoma, lymphoma, and pyogenic organisms (staph, strep).

11. Here is a partial list of causes of pulmonary nodules:

LEAVE THAT CHEST ALONE PLEASE

Lung cancer
Embolism
Aspirated foreign body
Vasculitis
Echinococcus

Tumor metastasis
Heart worm
Amyloidoma
Tuberculosis

Coccidioides and other fungal diseases
Hamartoma
Enlarged pulmonary artery
Sarcoidosis
Teratoma

Arteriovenous malformation
Lymphoma
Organizing pneumonia/BOOP
Necrobiotic nodules (rheumatoid arthritis)
Eosinophilic granuloma

Pseudotumor
Localized anthrosilicosis
Endothelial tumor (hemangiopericytoma)
Atelectasis (round)
Sequestration
Erythrocytes (hematoma)

REFRACTORY HYPOTENSION

CRASHING

Cardiovascular
Respiratory
Addison's/Acidosis
Sepsis/toxic
Hypocalcemia
Inaccurate reading
Neurologic
GI bleed/internal bleeding

Notes

1. Although there are many causes of hypotension, when *refractory* hypotension is encountered, you must consider a very specific list of possible etiologies.

Turn to this list when a patient's blood pressure fails to increase despite use of intravenous fluids or pressor agents. Many of these causes of refractory hypotension are emergencies and require urgent treatment.

2. A simple system for remembering the causes of refractory hypotension is summarized by the mnemonic CRASHING, or by the mnemonic TERMINAL—Toxic/drugs, Endocrine/electrolytes, Respiratory, Myocardial/vascular, Infection/sepsis, Neurologic, Artifact, Losing blood.

3. **Cardiovascular** causes include right ventricular infarction, pulmonary embolism, cardiac tamponade, arrythmia, and massive left ventricular infarction. **Respiratory** causes often are seen in patients on the ventilator and include tension pneumothorax and auto-PEEP, which occurs when patients are over-ventilated or have severe airway obstruction. Endocrine causes include **Addison's** disease, and systemic **acidosis** may cause hypotension. **Sepsis/toxic** causes include bacterial septic shock, toxic shock, anaphylaxis, and drug overdose. **Hypocalcemia** may cause hypotension since vascular tone and pressor agents are calcium dependent. **Inaccurate blood pressure readings** may result from poor blood pressure cuff fit, peripheral vascular disease, and venous obstruction (e.g., superior vena cava syndrome), leading to a false impression of refractory hypotension. **Neurologic** causes include CVA, spinal cord injury, and epidural anesthesia. **GI bleeding** may be occult, or blood loss may occur in the thorax, retroperitoneal area, or abdomen.

4. The following mnemonic lists specific causes of refractory hypotension:

ALARM, BP THAT'S DROPPING

Artifact (poor cuff fit, peripheral vascular disease,
   superior vena cava syndrome)
Liver failure
Arrhythmia
Right ventricular infarct
Massive left ventricular infarct

Blood transfusion
Pulmonary embolism

Tamponade
Hypocalcemia
Addison's
Tension pneumothorax
Sepsis

Drugs/toxins (anaphylaxis, drug overdose, snake venom)
Rewarming hypothermia
Occult blood loss
Pancreatitis
PEEP/auto-PEEP
Intubation (usually transient)
Neurogenic (spinal cord injury, epidural anesthesia, dysautonomia)
Gastrointestinal bleeding

SARCOIDOSIS

HILAR NODES*

Hepatosplenomegaly
Interstitial fibrosis, pulmonary
Lymphadenopathy
Arthralgia/arthritis
Renal (calcium metabolism abnormalities, nephrolithiasis)

Neurologic involvement (unilateral facial paralysis, chronic meningitis, mass lesion)
Ophthalmologic (uveitis, conjunctival granulomas, sicca syndrome)
Diabetes insipidus/other pituitary deficiency
Erythema nodosum/other skin lesion
Salivary gland enlargement, bilateral

* Clinical characteristics

SARCOID BLUES**

Skin rash
Arthropathy/arthralgias
Respiratory
Central nervous system
Optic (uveitis, iritis)
Incidental finding on chest x-ray
Dysrhythmia/cardiac dysfunction

Bone marrow/spleen
Lofgren's syndrome (erythema nodosum, fever,
    malleolar, join pain, hilar adenopathy)
Uveoparotid fever (e.g., Heerfordt's syndrome)
Ear, nose, and throat
Systemic symptoms (fever, chills, myalgias,
    hypercalcemia)

** *Possible presentations*

Notes

1. Sarcoidosis is a multisystem disease. Virtually any organ system may be involved.
   - Pulmonary interstitial involvement (up to 100%)
   - Lymphadenopathy, hilar/mediastinal (75–90%)
   - Arthralgia/arthritis (25–50%)
   - Bone marrow (15–40%), but rarely symptomatic beyond mild anemia, neutropenia, and eosinophilia
   - Hepatomegaly/liver enzyme elevation (20–30%)
   - Ophthalmologic (25%): uveitis (75–95% of eye cases)
   - Erythema nodosum (25%), skin lesions
   - Upper respiratory tract (up to 20%)
   - Salivary gland, parotid enlargement, bilateral (10%)
   - Splenomegaly (5–10%)
   - Neurologic involvement (5%): unilateral facial paralysis (most common), papilledema, hearing abnormal, hypothalamic/pituitary lesion, chronic meningitis, mass lesion, seizure
   - Cardiac disease (5%): arrhythmias, heart block, pericarditis, CHF
   - Renal: calcium metabolism abnormal, nephrolithiasis (rare, < 5%)
   - Diabetes insipidus or other pituitary deficiency

2. Pulmonary, ocular, lymph node, and skin changes are the most common, clinically important features.

3. Many cases are found incidentally on chest x-ray. In fact, this is one of only a few diseases in which a patient may have a markedly abnormal chest x-ray, but appear quite healthy.

4. The disease pathogenesis may be related to exaggerated helper T-cell activity.

5. Hypercalcemia is due to an increase in 1,25-hydroxylase activity in the granulomas. It often responds to steroid therapy.

6. Certain factors are associated with progressive disease in sarcoidosis, the presence of which may be reason for more aggressive initial therapy. These factors include chronic uveitis, chronic bone disease, nephrocalcinosis, skin plaques, lupus pernio, and pulmonary infiltrates without nodules ("type 3" pulmonary sarcoidosis).

▦

HEMATOLOGY

General Considerations

The differential diagnosis for a hematologic disorder can be developed using the MEDICINE DOC categories:

Metabolic (e.g., amyloidosis, B12 and folate deficiencies)

Endocrine (e.g., paraneoplastic syndromes, adrenal insufficiency, hypothyroidism)

Drugs/medicines (e.g., antibiotics, alcohol, chemotherapy toxicity)

Infection (e.g., HIV-related, TB, systemic infections)

Congenital (e.g., Fanconi's, chronic granulomatous disease, protein C deficiency)

Immunologic (e.g., hemolytic anemia, ITP, autoimmune neutropenia)

Neoplastic (e.g., leukemia, lymphoma, metastatic disease)

Exotic diseases (e.g., sarcoid, porphyria, Wegener's)

Degenerative (?myelodysplasia; also premalignant)

Occupational/environmental (e.g., radiation, hydrocarbons, heavy metal poisoning)

Cardiovascular (e.g., intracardiac shunt, hypercoagulable states causing DVT/PE)

Problems considered in the hematology section primarily involve the bone marrow and often are made manifest by a decrease or increase in one of the primary blood cell types: RBCs, WBCs, and platelets. Also included are abnormalities of the spleen and disorders of coagulation.

ANEMIA

MCVS

Marrow problem
Consumption/destruction
Volume increase (hemodilution)
Stool/menstrual/occult losses

Notes

1. Anemia is defined as a drop in the hemoglobin concentration. The four basic mechanisms are listed above. Examination of the peripheral smear and red cell indices (i.e., mean cell volume [MCV], RBC distribution width) is the first step in evaluation of anemia. The MCV is the most helpful index to guide the work-up. The mnemonic "MCVS" helps to narrow down the differential by classifying an anemia as microcytic, normocytic, or macrocytic.

2. **Marrow problems** are characterized by a decrease in production of RBCs. There may be a deficiency in components needed for normal RBC synthesis; the marrow may be invaded and replaced by an infiltrative process such as a malignancy ("myelophthisic process"); or there may be primary marrow dysfunction ("myelodysplasia"). Marrow problems may be microcytic (i.e., processes that perturb hemoglobin production, such as iron deficiency), normocytic (i.e., myelodysplasia), or macrocytic (i.e., processes that interfere with RBC maturation, such as B12 deficiency).

3. **Consumption/destruction** of erythrocytes occurs in patients with autoimmune or neoplastic diseases (hemolytic anemia), mechanical heart valves, severe systemic illnesses such as sepsis (DIC), or thrombotic thrombocytopenic purpura (TTP). RBCs are destroyed either by antibodies (autoimmune disorders) or an intravascular cause (mechanical heart valve or blood vessel process). Intravascular injury is called "microangiopathic," and the peripheral smear features damaged RBCs called "schistocytes." Consumptive/destructive processes are accompanied by increased bone marrow activity and more reticulocytes in the peripheral smear. Since the reticulocyte is a young, large RBC, there is an

increase in the MCV. Thus these processes usually are macrocytic, unless there is concomitant marrow failure (i.e., iron deficiency from chronic hemolysis).

4. **Volume increase** causes hemodilution and a decrease in hemoglobin concentration. This situation is encountered when dehydrated patients receive intravenous fluids. Also, in acute blood loss, intravenous fluids may make the blood loss manifest since the initial hemoglobin may be normal. The MCV is unaffected by volume increase and is usually normocytic.

5. **Stool/menstrual/occult blood losses** frequently are accompanied by iron deficiency and are common causes of microcytic anemia. Young women are often anemic because of monthly menstrual blood loss. The other common cause of blood loss is occult GI bleeding leading to hemoccult positive stools. Less commonly, occult blood loss occurs from an internal source, such as a retroperitoneal bleed. Retroperitoneal bleeding may occur after an invasive procedure or as a complication of anticoagulation. In addition to a drop in the hemoglobin, the BUN increases from absorbed heme metabolites.

6. The mnemonic below divides the anemias into categories according to the MCV: microcytic, normocytic, or macrocytic.

IT'S ANEMIA'S BRAND

Microcytic
Iron deficiency
Thalassemia
Sideroblastic anemia

Usually Normocytic
Anemia of chronic disease
Nephrogenic anemia (uremia)
Endocrine disorders
Myelophthisis (marrow infiltration)
IV fluids
Aplastic anemia
Sickle cell anemia

Usually Macrocytic
B12 deficiency
Reticulocytosis/hemolysis
Alcohol/cirrhosis
Nutritional deficiency (folate)
Drugs (**D**NA synthesis inhibitors, **D**ihydrofolate reductase inhibitors)

7. Microcytic anemias are due to a deficiency of one of the three major constituents of hemoglobin: iron, globin, and porphyrin. Hemoglobin comprises 90% of the protein in the RBC, so microcytic cells are small and pale. **Iron deficiency** is seen in states of chronic blood loss (stool, menstrual, occult), RBC destruction (hemolysis), or nutritional deficiency (vegetarian diet). The **thalassemias** are a diverse group of diseases resulting in defective globin chain production. The **sideroblastic anemias** are characterized by "ringed sideroblasts" in the marrow and abnormal porphyrin synthesis. They may be hereditary (rare, X-linked), acquired (alcohol, isoniazid, lead), or idiopathic (premalignant).

8. Normocytic anemia is seen in many disease states. The **anemia of chronic disease** is seen whenever there is long-standing inflammation or systemic disease. It is characterized by low serum iron and total iron-binding capacity, but an elevated or normal serum ferritin. **Nephrogenic anemia** is caused by reduced erythropoetin levels and can be ameliorated by erythropoetin replacement therapy. **Endocrine disorders** often feature a normocytic anemia because many hormones affect RBC proliferation, including thyroxine, glucocorticoids, testosterone, and growth hormone. Less commonly, hypothyroidism causes macrocytosis. **Myelophthisis** is marrow infiltration by neoplasm, infection, or metabolic disease (neoplasms can cause anemia by a variety of mechanisms, including myelophthisis, hemolytic anemia, occult blood loss, nutritional deficiency, or the effects of chemotherapy). Myelophthisic processes cause a normocytic anemia, and the peripheral smear may show immature erythroid forms and, occasionally, marked neutrophilia ("leukemoid reaction"). **Intravenous fluids** cause a dilutional decrease in hemoglobin concentration and may unmask anemia after acute blood loss. **Aplastic anemia** may be a primary marrow failure or secondary to drug toxicity. **Sickle cell anemia**, a hemoglobinopathy, features abnormally shaped cells, but the MCV is usually normal.

9. Macrocytic anemias are usually a result of an impairment of DNA replication. Often the LDH level is very high due to accelerated turnover in the marrow or peripherally. **B12 (cobalamin) deficiency** can occur in several settings, including gastrointestinal disease, chronic nitrous oxide use, and, rarely, nutritional deficiency. Both B12 and folate are important cofactors in DNA synthesis, and a deficiency in either results in large, abnormal RBCs. Macrocytosis also occurs with RBC destruction (e.g., hemolytic anemia, TTP) because of compensatory **reticulocytosis** (see above).

Alcohol depresses bone marrow RBC production, causing anemia, often macrocytic. Alcoholics may have primary macrocytosis (usually modest) or secondary macrocytosis from folate and/or B12 deficiency. Anemia in cirrhotic patients may be microcytic, normocytic, or macrocytic because of their myriad problems including blood loss, nutritional deficiency, and the effects of chronic disease. Less commonly, cirrhotics have a hemolytic anemia called spur cell anemia that is caused by the abnormal lipoprotein balance present in advanced liver disease. The diagnosis is made when a cirrhotic patient has evidence of hemolysis with characteristic "spur" cells in the peripheral smear.

Nutritional deficiency of folate is seen in starvation, conditions with increased requirements (pregnancy, malignancy, chronic hemolysis, chronic exfoliative skin diseases, hemodialysis), and malabsorption. **Drugs** that inhibit **dihydrolate reductase** (e.g., methotrexate, triamterene) or **DNA metabolism** (e.g., 5-FU, hydroxyurea, azathioprine, AZT, acyclovir) also cause a macrocytic anemia.

10. The work-up of anemia includes ruling out occult blood loss (usually stool or menstrual), examination of the peripheral smear, checking for deficiencies (iron, folate, or B12), a reticulocyte count to assess marrow activity, a hemolysis work-up (bilirubin, LDH, haptoglobin, serum free hemoglobin), and possibly a bone marrow biopsy.

11. The reticulocyte count is an indication of the marrow's capacity to make RBCs. Here is a slightly different mnemonic for anemia (still based on MCV) that emphasizes the importance of the reticulocyte count:

IT'S A RETICS DEFECT

Microcytic
Iron deficiency
Thalassemia
Sideroblastic anemia

Usually Normocytic
Aplastic anemia

Renal failure
Endocrine disorders
Tumor/myelophthisis
Illness/**I**nflammation (chronic disease)
Cirrhosis (may cause macrocytosis or spur cell anemia)
Sickle cell anemia

Usually Macrocytic
Drugs (**D**NA synthesis inhibitors, **D**ihydrofolate reductase inhibitors)
EtOH
Folate
Erythroleukemia (Di Guglielmo's)
Cobalamin deficiency (B12)
TTP/hemolysis

BLEEDING DIATHESES

APTT

Anatomic abnormality (e.g., AVM, peptic ulcer)
Plasma protein abnormality
Thrombocytopenia/qualitative platelet abnormality
Trauma

Notes

1. A bleeding problem is most commonly related to an **anatomic abnormality**. Congenital abnormalities such as an arteriovenous malformation or acquired defects such as peptic ulcer disease are common. **Plasma protein abnormalities** are less common and may be made manifest with unexpected hemorrhage associated with a minor surgical procedure. **Thrombocytopenia** has many causes and is relatively common, but **qualitative platelet abnormalities** are rare. Finally, **trauma** is a common cause of hemorrhage and usually obvious, but excessive bleeding or bruising after minor trauma may indicate an occult bleeding diathesis.
2. The **APTT**, PT, platelet count, and bleeding time are the primary laboratory studies obtained when investigating a possible plasma protein abnormality or qualitative platelet defect. Other tests including thrombin time, fibrinogen assay, clot solubility and lysis, and factor assays may be helpful in identifying specific deficiencies.

Primary Hemostatic (Platelet) Disorders

Platelet adhesion defects:
    Von Willebrand's disease
    Bernard-Soulier syndrome (absence, dysfunction of Gplb/IX)
Platelet aggregation defects
    Glanzmann's thrombasthenia (absence, dysfunction of Gpllb/llla)
Platelet release defects

- Decreased cyclooxygenase activity
  Drugs—aspirin, nonsteroidal anti-inflammatory agents
  Congenital
- Granule storage pool defects
  Congenital
  Acquired
- Uremia
- Platelet coating (e.g., penicillin or paraproteins)

Platelet coagulant defect
    Scott's syndrome

Gp = glycoprotein.

Relationship Between Secondary Hemostatic Disorders and Coagulation Test Abnormalities

Prolonged partial thromboplastin time (PTT)
    No clinical bleeding—factors XII, HMWK, PK
    Mild or rare bleeding—factor XI
    Frequent, severe bleeding—factors VIII and IX
Prolonged prothrombin time (PT)
    Factor VII deficiency
    Vitamin K deficiency—early
    Warfarin anticoagulant ingestion
Prolonged PTT and PT
    Factor II, V, or X deficiency
    Vitamin K deficiency—late
    Warfarin anticoagulant ingestion
Prolonged thrombin time (TT)
    Mild or rare bleeding—afibrinogenemia
    Frequent, severe bleeding—dysfibrinogenemia
    Heparin-like inhibitors or heparin administration
Prolonged PT and/or PTT not corrected with normal plasma
    Specific or nonspecific inhibitor syndromes
Clot solubility in 5 M urea
    Factor XIII deficiency
    Inhibitors or defective cross-linking
Rapid clot lysis
    Alpha$_2$ plasmin inhibitor

HMWK = high-molecular-weight kininogen; PK = prekallikrein.

Both tables from Handin RI: Bleeding and thrombosis. In Isselbacher KJ, et al (eds): Harrison's Principles of Internal Medicine, 13th ed. New York, McGraw-Hill, Inc., 1994, pp 317–322; with permission.

SPLENOMEGALY

BANTI'S

Blood flow problem
Anemia/erythrocyte problem
Neoplasm/infiltrative disease
Thyrotoxicosis
Infection
Sarcoid/**S**ystemic lupus erythematosus

Notes

1. **Banti's** syndrome is the eponym used to describe congestive splenomegaly with hypersplenism. Using "BANTI'S" as your guide, the causes of spleno-megaly can be classified in six categories. **Blood flow problems** cause spleno-megaly by increased splenic vein pressures and consequent congestion. Splenic vein thrombosis (often secondary to pancreatitis), portal vein thrombosis or ex-trinsic compression, cirrhosis, hepatic vein thrombosis (Budd-Chiari syndrome), and CHF all cause congestive splenomegaly. **Anemias secondary to erythro-cyte abnormalities** (e.g., thalassemias, sickle cell disease, hereditary spherocy-tosis) cause splenomegaly because there is hyperplasia of the reticuloendothelial system associated with the destruction of the abnormal RBCs. These diseases also may cause splenic infarction (i.e., sickle cell).

    Neoplasms and infiltrative diseases directly involve the spleen and lead to its enlargement. In myeloproliferative syndromes and myelophthisic processes, because of marrow hypofunction, there may be compensatory extramedullary hematopoiesis causing splenomegaly. **Thyrotoxicosis** is associated with splenomegaly because of thyroid hormone–induced lymphoid hyperplasia. Numerous **infections**, usually chronic, may cause splenomegaly. Disorders of immune regulation such as **sarcoidosis and SLE** may feature splenomegaly. Other examples include rheumatoid arthritis (Felty's syndrome), serum sickness, and immune hemolytic anemias.

2. The degree of splenomegaly varies with the disease entity. Massive splenomegaly occurs in chronic myelocytic leukemia, myelofibrosis with myeloid metaplasia, hairy cell leukemia, Gaucher's and Niemann-Pick diseases, sar-coidosis, thalassemia major, chronic malaria, congenital syphilis, leishmaniasis, and some cases of portal vein obstruction. These are chronic diseases in which the spleen slowly enlarges. Rupture of the spleen may be seen in acute infec-tious processes such as EBV mononucleosis, malaria, and typhoid fever.

3. Here is a more comprehensive listing of the causes of splenomegaly:

HIS BIG SPLENIC MASS

Hepatic vein obstruction (Budd-Chiari)
Infection
Splenic vein thrombosis (e.g., pancreatitis)

Berylliosis
Infiltrative diseases (e.g., Gaucher's, amyloid,
   eosinophilic granulomatosis)
Grave's disease/hyperthyroidism

SLE/collagen vascular diseases
Portal vein obstruction
Liver disease (cirrhosis)
Erythrocyte abnormality (e.g., spherocytosis, sickle cell, thalassemia)
Neoplasm (lymphoma, myeloproliferative disease, metastatic)
Iron deficiency
CHF (congestive splenomegaly)

Myeloproliferative disease
Autoimmune-hemolytic anemia
Sarcoidosis
Serum sickness/drug reaction

4. Always consider an occult, infectious etiology for splenomegaly since these diseases are likely to respond to appropriate therapy. There are numerous infections associated with splenomegaly, many of which are listed in Chapter IV (see "Infections Causing Splenomegaly").

Clinical Conditions or Diagnoses

EOSINOPHILIA

ALLERGIC

Addison's (adrenal insufficiency)
Lymphoma/malignancy
L-tryptophan
Eczema/skin diseases
Respiratory diseases (asthma, allergic bronchopulmonary aspergillosis, PIE syndromes)
Gastroenteritis
Infections (helminths, coccidioides mycosis)
Collagen vascular diseases

Notes

1. Eosinophilia is defined as > 500 eosinophils/microliter of blood. Eosinophilia has diverse disease associations, but "ALLERGIC" reactions are probably the most common. Allergic reactions to drugs, pollens, micro-organisms, and other antigens can stimulate eosinophilia.

2. **Addison's** disease frequently features a moderate eosinophilia that resolves with administration of corticosteroids. **Lymphoma** is the malignancy most commonly associated with eosinophilia, although associations with many solid tumors have been described. Tumor-associated eosinophilia is probably a result of interleukin-5 secretion and often indicates a widely disseminated tumor. Eosinophilic leukemia is a rare hematologic neoplasm with dramatically high eosinophil counts. **L-tryptophan** preparations from a single source were implicated in the eosinophilia-myalgia syndrome, a potentially fatal, multisystem disease. **Eczema** and several other skin diseases (e.g., pemphigus, mycosis fungoides) may be associated with eosinophilia.

Several **respiratory diseases** feature eosinophilia, including asthma and the PIE (pulmonary infiltrates with eosinophilia) syndromes. The PIE syndromes include acute eosinophilic pneumonia, chronic eosinophilic pneumonia, Churg-Strauss vasculitis, parasitic infestation (i.e., "tropical" pneumonia), and allergic bronchopulmonary aspergillosis (ABPA). The hypereosinophilic syndrome, a multisystem disease, may cause eosinophilic infiltration of any organ including the lungs. Drugs also can cause eosinophilia with pulmonary infiltration.

Eosinophilic **gastroenteritis** is characterized by eosinophilic infiltration of any portion of the gastrointestinal tract, peripheral eosinophilia (75% of cases), and inflammatory diarrhea. **Infections** with helminths typically cause eosinophilia, and coccidioides mycosis is unique among fungal infections in its propensity to elicit eosinophilia. **Collagen vascular diseases** such as rheumatoid arthritis, eosinophilic fasciitis, allergic angiitis, sarcoidosis, and Wegener's granulomatosis also are associated with eosinophilia.

3. The eponym **Löeffler's** has been applied to PIE syndromes, the idiopathic hypereosinophilic syndrome, and to eosinophilic endocarditis. Löeffler originally described transient pulmonary infiltrates with eosinophilia, which may have been related to ascariasis infestation. Although it has no specific definition, the name is still used in cases of idiopathic, benign pulmonary infiltrates with eosinophilia.

4. The cytokine IL-5 is an important stimulator of eosinophils and is probably integral in many or all causes of eosinophilia. The following mnemonic, emphasizing the role of IL-5, lists the causes of eosinophilia:

PLASMA IL-FIVE RAGE

Parasites
L-tryptophan
Addison's
Sarcoidosis
Malignancy (e.g., Hodgkin's, CML, gastric, ovarian, lung, pancreatic cancers)
Allergy/**A**topy (e.g., drugs, serum sickness, hay fever)

Idiopathic hypereosinophilic syndrome
Lung diseases/Löeffler's

Fungal (ABPA, coccidioides mycosis)
IgE hypersecretion (Job's syndrome)
Vasculitis/collagen vascular disease
Eczema/skin diseases

Recovery from bone marrow transplant
Angiogram/**A**theromatous emboli ("cholesterol emboli")
Gastroenteritis
Endomyocardial

ERYTHROCYTOSIS

HI RBCS

Hypoxia/hypoventilation
Inappropriate erythropoietin

Relative polycythemia (stress, dehydration)
Bone marrow disorder
Carboxyhemoglobin/congenital hemoglobinopathies
Steroids/androgens

Notes

1. Erythrocytosis or polycythemia indicates an increase in number of erythrocytes in a sample of blood, which may or may not be a reflection of total body red cells. It is important to distinguish between *absolute erythrocytosis,* a true increase in total body red cell mass, and *relative erythrocytosis,* which occurs with dehydration (increase in RBC concentration) and stress.
2. The basic mechanisms of erythrocytosis are summarized by "HI RBCS."

HYPERCOAGULABLE STATES

PT INRS

Platelets
Trauma

Immobolization/stasis
Neoplasm
RBCs
Serum clotting factors

Notes

1. Numerous disorders may predispose patients to thrombosis. Frequently, the history and physical examination reveal a likely etiology. Factors predisposing to thrombosis include obesity, varicose veins, trauma, general anesthesia, immobilization, malignancy, CHF, oral contraceptives, infection, pregnancy, nephrotic syndrome, and blood protein defects.
2. Leiden factor 5, a mutation in which factor 5 is resistant to activated protein C, is the most common inherited hypercoagulable condition known. Homozygous individuals are at high risk for recurrent thromboembolic events. The risk for heterozygotes is less clear.

3. Protein deficiencies may be difficult to identify. Current tests only identify 10–20% of the cases of familial thrombosis. Serum levels of proteins C and S will be affected by large thrombi and warfarin anticoagulation. Deficiencies may be congenital or acquired. Antithrombin (AT)-III, protein C, and protein S are the most common congenital conditions. The most common acquired defects are AT-III and antiphospholipid antibodies.

4. The "lupus anticoagulant" is an antiphospholipid antibody that prolongs the PTT by interfering with phospholipid in the laboratory assay. It does not cause clinical bleeding, but rather predisposes to thrombosis and mid-trimester abortion.

5. Urinary AT-III loss probably causes hypercoagulability in patients with the nephrotic syndrome. These patients are predisposed to renal vein thrombosis and pulmonary embolism.

6. High levels of homocystine predispose patients to arterial as well as venous thrombosis. Homocystine also may be an important factor in the development of atherosclerosis.

7. An important drug-related cause of hypercoagulability is heparin-associated thrombocytopenia. The features are arterial thrombosis with falling platelet counts. Even low doses of subcutaneous heparin can cause this syndrome. A heparin-aggregation study is available for laboratory confirmation in suspected cases.

8. Here is a more comprehensive list of hypercoagulable states:

DVT, PE AND CLOTS

Drugs (e.g., tamoxifen, heparin)
Venous catheter (central)
Trauma (endothelial injury)

Prosthetic valves
Erythrocytosis (polycythemia)

Anticardiolipin/**A**ntiphospholipid antibodies
Nephrotic syndrome/**N**eoplasm
Dysfunctional platelets/**D**ysfibrogenemia

CHF/**C**ollagen vascular disease (e.g., Behçet's, SLE)
Leiden factor V/**L**ow protein C and S
Obstetrics/**O**ral contraceptives
TTP/**T**hromboangiitis obliterans
Smoking/**S**tasis

Also: hyperviscosity (Waldenstrom's), homocystinuria, AT-III, alpha-1 antiplasmin, heparin cofactor II, plasminogen, plasminogen activator, and factor XII deficiencies.

LYMPHOPENIA

NOT A T CELL

Normal variant/no disease
Occult carcinoma
TB/infections

AIDS

Thoracic duct drainage/chylothorax

Cytotoxic drugs/chemotherapy
Eating disorder/malnutrition
Lymphoma
Lupus/collagen vascular disease

Notes

1. *Absolute lymphopenia* is defined as < 1000 lymphocytes/ml. *Relative lymphopenia* is present when < 15% of leukocytes are lymphocytes. Absolute lymphopenia is most often secondary to steroid therapy or cytotoxic drugs, but the literature suggests numerous disease associations. In truth, any severe systemic illness may feature lymphopenia.

2. Although the disease associations are myriad, the finding of lymphopenia is important because it is relatively rare. In one, pre-AIDS era study of patients at a major referral center, the incidence of either absolute or relative lymphopenia was only 2.4%, and it was significantly associated with malignancy. Given the increased severity of illness in this referral group of patients, it is probable that the incidence of lymphopenia in the general population is much less.

3. The consequences of lymphopenia include life-threatening infections, especially those caused by viruses, fungi, and mycobacteria. Since lymphocytes are important in immune surveillance and preventing neoplastic proliferation, lymphopenia also may predispose patients to malignancies. As mentioned above, there is an association between lymphopenia and malignancy, but cause and effect are not certain.

4. Lymphopenia may be a clue to an underlying systemic disease such as AIDS, lupus, or lymphoma. Consider the possibility of AIDS in any patient with unexplained lymphopenia. In addition to the diseases listed below, lymphopenia has been seen in patients with COPD, drug allergy, advanced age,

hyperparathyroidism, trigeminal neuralgia, myasthenia gravis (without thymectomy), periodic paralysis, amyotrophic lateral sclerosis, and hypothyroidism.

I'M HELPLESS WITHOUT T AND B CELLS

Irradiation
Malaria

Heart failure
Electrocution/burns
Lymphocyte antiglobulin therapy
Pancreatitis
Lupus
Exhaustion
Steroids
Starvation (pyridoxine deficiency)

Whipple's disease
Infection/sepsis
TB
Hereditary immunodeficiencies
Occult carcinoma
Uremia
Thymectomy

Thoracic duct drainage

AIDS
Normal variant/no disease
Diabetes

Bone marrow failure (agranulocytosis)

Chemotherapy/cytotoxic drugs
Extracorporeal blood irradiation
Lymphoma
Liver failure
Sarcoidosis

MONOCYTOSIS

MONO

Mycobacteria
Other odd infections
Neoplasm (metastatic)
Other inflammatory conditions

Notes

1. Monocytes are circulating cells with a half-life of 12–24 hours. They leave the blood stream and enter tissues, differentiating into macrophages ("big eaters") specific for the particular organ (e.g., alveolar macrophages, splenic macrophages, liver Kupffer cells, brain microglial cells, dendritic cells). They have diverse functions, such as phagocytosis, lymphocyte activation, and other cytokine-mediated activities. Many disorders affecting PMNs, including toxins and infections, also affect monocytes. A significant increase in monocytes, however, should prompt consideration of certain specific conditions.
2. In the presence of monocytosis, examine for malignancy, tuberculosis, and a few other odd infections.
3. Here is a more specific differential for monocytosis, emphasizing the evolution of a peripheral blood monocyte into a tissue-specific macrophage:

I'LL BE A MACROPHAGE

Inflammatory bowel disease
Leukemia
Leishmaniasis (kala azar)

Brucellosis
Endocarditis

Arteritis (polyarteritis nodosa, temporal arteritis)

Myeloproliferative disorders
Acid-fast bacilli (TB, other mycobacteria)
Cytomegalovirus
Rocky Mountain spotted fever
Oncologic/**O**ccult malignancy (usually metastatic
disease)
Plasmodium infections (malaria)
Hemolytic anemia
Acquired neutrophil disorders (e.g., chronic
granulomatous disease, Chediak-Higashi)
Granulomatous diseases (sarcoid, berylliosis)
Evan's syndrome

NEUTROPENIA

ANCS

Autoimmune/**A**ntibodies
Neoplasm/infiltrative/toxic
Cardiopulmonary bypass/hemodialysis
Sepsis/overwhelming infection

N otes

1. The normal concentration of neutrophils is approximately 3650/ml (range 1830–7250). The absolute neutrophil count ("ANC") is determined by multiplying the percent neutrophils by the total white blood cell count. When the ANC is less than 1000, infectious complications increase significantly, and the inflammatory process is essentially absent when the ANC is less than 200. Neutropenia may result from four basic mechanisms: autoimmune or antibody-mediated peripheral destruction; neoplastic, infiltrative, or toxic depression of the marrow; cardiopulmonary bypass and hemodialysis; or sepsis/overwhelming infection.

2. **Autoimmune processes** may feature **antineutrophil antibodies** and/or hypersplenism, causing neutropenia. Examples include SLE, rheumatoid arthritis, Felty's syndrome, and Wegener's granulomatosis. Drugs such as diuretics,

alpha-methyl dopa, and some phenothiazines also may act as haptens, promoting peripheral destruction of neutrophils.

3. Processes that impair marrow production of neutrophils include **neoplastic invasion, infiltrative/infectious involvement of the marrow**, and the **cytotoxic effects of drugs.** Neutropenia is common in patients treated with high doses of chemotherapy. The duration and severity of neutropenia can be ameliorated by administration of G-CSF.

4. Cardiopulmonary bypass and **hemodialysis** cause peripheral pooling and a transient neutropenia. **Sepsis/overwhelming infections** also may cause a transient neutropenia, which may be an effect of endotoxin release. Be careful not to miss sepsis, especially in elderly patients, who may have a paucity of other signs of infection.

5. Neutropenic patients are predisposed to infections with bacteria and fungi (especially *Candida* and *Aspergillus*). Some conditions occurring predominantly in neutropenic patients include skin lesions from fungal infection, ecthyma gangrenosum (often a result of *Pseudomonas* infection). Sweet's syndrome (neutrophilic dermatosis), typhlitis (inflammation of the cecum), perirectal infections, and opportunistic pneumonias.

6. Here is a more complete differential for neutropenia:

MINIMAL White Blood CellS

Medications/toxins (especially chemotherapy)
Idiopathic (benign cyclic neutropenia)
Nutritional (B12, folate)
Infection (e.g., sepsis, mononucleosis, typhoid)
Myelophthisis/invasion of marrow
Aplastic anemia
Leukemia

Wegener's
Benign cyclic neutropenia
Chediak-Higashi/**C**ongenital neutropenias
Splenomegaly

NEUTROPHILIA

PMNS

Peripheral demargination
Marrow release
New synthesis
Systemic disease/miscellaneous

Notes

1. Neutrophilia, an increase in "PMNS" (polymorphonuclear neutrophils), results from four primary processes: peripheral demargination of existing PMNs, marrow release of an existing pool of PMNs, newly synthesized PMNs, and stimulation by miscellaneous systemic diseases (probably by a combination of related processes).

2. **Peripheral demargination** occurs when neutrophils outside the bone marrow are released from their sites of adherence along blood vessels (many along vessels in the spleen and lung). This process can rapidly double the number of neutrophils seen on the peripheral smear. Demargination occurs with physiologic stress, exercise, exogenous epinephrine administration, steroid therapy, and nonsteroidal anti-inflammatory agents. The deficiency of the leukocyte adhesion protein CR3 causes neutrophils to adhere poorly to endothelial cells and margination is inhibited. Patients with this defect have prominent neutrophilia and recurrent infections.

3. **Marrow release** of an existing pool of neutrophils occurs with steroid therapy, acute infections, and inflammation (e.g., thermal injury).

4. **New synthesis of PMNs** occurs in response to infections, necrosis of tissue (e.g., gangrene, pulmonary or myocardial infarction, thermal injury), inflammatory states (e.g., vasculitis, hypersensitivity reactions), steroid therapy, and myeloproliferative disorders (e.g., polycythemia vera, AML, myeloid metaplasia).

5. Various systemic disorders, including diabetic ketoacidosis, uremia from acute renal failure, metastatic cancers, acute hemorrhage, hemolysis, and eclampsia, can stimulate neutrophilia. Toxic exposures such as poisoning and lithium administration also may be associated with neutrophilia. The mechanism of neutrophilia in these disorders may be a combination of the above processes.

6. Persistent neutrophilia of 30,000 to 50,000 cells/ml is called a **leukemoid reaction** (to distinguish from leukemia) and may be the result of malignant

invasion of bone marrow, extensive inflammation, or severe infection. The neutrophils seen in the circulation are usually mature.

7. Two more specific differentials for neutrophilia are given below:

HI PMNS

Hemorrhage
Infection

Physiologic (stress)
Myeloproliferative disorder
Necrosis of tissue
Steroids

Note: This mnemonic emphasizes the most common etiologies of neutrophilia.

MAD NEUTROPHILS

Myeloproliferative disorder
Adhesion protein deficiency (leukocyte CR3 receptor)
Diabetic ketoacidosis

Necrosis of tissue
Eclampsia
Uremia (acute renal failure)
Toxin ingestion
Rheumatologic disorders/vasculitis
Oncologic (usually metastatic)
Physiologic (stress)
Hemorrhage/**H**emolysis
Infection
Lithium
Steroids

Note: This mnemonic lists most of the causes of neutrophilia.

PANCYTOPENIA

AIDS?

Aplastic marrow
Invaded marrow
Dysplastic marrow
Splenomegaly

N otes

1. There are four primary mechanisms of pancytopenia: aplastic marrow (hypocellular), invaded marrow (neoplasm, storage diseases), dysplastic marrow (normo or hypercellular), and splenomegaly. As the mnemonic suggests, HIV infection should be considered in any patient with pancytopenia.
2. Causes of **aplastic** anemia include congenital disorders (e.g., Fanconi's anemia), chemical and other toxic exposures (e.g., benzene, alkylating agents, arsenicals, radiation), immunologically mediated aplasia (e.g., SLE), infections (e.g., hepatitis, parvovirus), other miscellaneous associations (e.g., pregnancy, transfusion-associated graft versus host disease), and idiopathic aplastic anemia. Marrow **invasion** and replacement occurs with hematologic malignancies, metastatic cancers, storage cell disorders, osteopetrosis, and myelofibrosis. **Dysplastic** disorders feature a normal or hypercellular marrow and include B12 deficiency, folate deficiency, AIDS, and primary myelodysplasia. Splenomegaly and consequent hypersplenism promote accelerated removal of cells from circulation, and marrow cellularity is usually normal.
3. In approaching pancytopenia, first rule out drugs, toxins, infections (e.g., AIDS), and nutritional deficiencies as causes. Examination of the peripheral smear may provide clues to the diagnosis, but bone marrow aspiration and biopsy are the definitive tests.
4. The following mnemonic lists the primary causes of pancytopenia:

LO PMNS AND RBCS

Leukemia
Osteopetrosis

Paroxysmal nocturnal hemoglobinuria
Myelodysplastic syndrome
Neoplastic invasion of bone marrow
Sarcoidosis

Aplastic anemic
Nutritional deficiency (B12, folate)
Drugs/toxins

Rheumatologic diseases
Big spleen
Congenital disease (Falconi's, Gaucher's)
Sepsis/infections

THROMBOTIC THROMBOCYTOPENIC PURPURA

RETIC

Renal dysfunction
Elevated temperature
Thrombocytopenia
Intravascular hemolysis
Central nervous system

Notes

1. TTP is a disease of unknown etiology. The diagnosis is based on the pentad of: (1) renal dysfunction, (2) elevated body temperature, (3) thrombocytopenia, (4) intravascular hemolysis ("microangiopathic"), and (5) central nervous system dysfunction (i.e., altered mental status, seizures).
2. TTP may be the result of endothelial release of **abnormal Von Willebrand factor multimers**. These multimers precipitate the formation of fibrin microthrombi

that occlude blood vessels and damage RBCs and platelets. There is also evidence that an inhibition or deficiency of a critical Von Willebrand cleaving factor is responsible for the microthrombi. The result is a microangiopathic process with severe thrombocytopenia and anemia. The primary end-organ damage is seen in renal and neurologic dysfunction. The peripheral smear is the key to making a prompt diagnosis and initiating treatment. The smear shows schistocytes, cells damaged by the microangiopathic process, and a marked reticulocytosis ("RETIC"). The reticulocytosis is evidence that the marrow is functioning normally in response to peripheral destruction of RBCs. The MCV (see Anemia section) is elevated because of the increase in these large, immature erythrocytes.

3. Coagulation tests are normal in TTP, whereas in DIC abnormalities of PT, PTT, fibrinogen, fibrin split products, and D-dimer are the rule.

4. Treatment of TTP involves prompt plasmapheresis and plasma exchange. Intravenous immunoglobulin, vincristine, and glucocorticoids may be beneficial, but controlled studies are lacking. Splenectomy may have a role in refractory cases. Platelet transfusions are not indicated.

5. Hemolytic uremic syndrome, a syndrome closely related to TTP, is seen predominantly in children and has more prominent renal involvement. It may occur after gastroenteritis caused by *E. coli* 0157:H7.

THROMBOCYTOPENIA

PLTS

Peripheral destruction
Lab error
Trapping (hypersplenism)
Synthesis problem (marrow failure)

Notes

1. Thrombocytopenia is a result of one of four problems: peripheral destruction, laboratory error, trapping in the spleen, and synthetic problems. **Peripheral destruction** of platelets occurs with ITP, DIC TTP, PTP, prosthetic valves, pregnancy-associated disorders, certain drugs, systemic infections, and collagen vascular diseases. **Laboratory error** may occur with automated differentials. Be certain to look at the peripheral smear to rule out platelet clumping, which will give a

falsely low count. **Trapping** in the spleen (sequestration) reduces circulating platelets and is seen in any of the processes that cause splenomegaly (see Splenomegaly section). **Synthesis problems** are primary bone marrow production abnormalities that occur with invasion of marrow, drugs (those causing marrow suppression), and some infections. Synthesis problems also may feature decreased numbers of other cells (see Pancytopenia section).

2. Acute thrombocytopenia is an emergency, and "ITPS" lists the most important etiologies. A prompt diagnosis is critical, because bleeding can be life-threatening, and the treatments differ.

ITPS

Idiopathic thrombocytopenic purpura (ITP)
Thrombotic thrombocytopenic purpura (TTP)
Pregnancy/**P**ost-transfusion purpura (PTP)
Sepsis/disseminated intravascular coagulation (DIC)

3. ITP or immune thrombocytopenia may occur as an isolated phenomenon or in association with malignancies, collagen vascular diseases, or administration of certain drugs. Antibody-mediated destruction of platelets may require immunosuppressive therapy. A careful search for a causative drug is critical, as small amounts of the offending agent can trigger the reaction. Prolonged thrombocytopenia occurs with drugs that are cleared slowly from the body, such as gold and phenytoin. Heparin causes a specific and potentially catastrophic syndrome of thrombocytopenia and arterial thrombosis called heparin-induced thrombocytopenia. The heparin-induced platelet antibody test is diagnostic. All heparin, including IV flushes, must be discontinued.

4. TTP and the closely related hemolytic uremic syndrome are treated with plasma exchange (see TTP section).

5. PTP and **pregnancy-associated syndromes** should be suspected in women with acute thrombocytopenia. PTP is a rare phenomenon that occurs 1 week after transfusion in individuals (almost always women) lacking certain platelet antigens (the most common is PLA1). Most patients have had a prior exposure to PLA1 antigens during pregnancy or a prior transfusion. Intravenous immunoglobulin or steroids may facilitate recovery in 4–5 days. The related pregnancy-associated syndromes of eclampsia, acute fatty liver, and HELLP (hemolysis with elevated liver enzymes and low platelets) are life-threatening. Microangiopathic destruction lowers platelets precipitously, and timely delivery of the fetus is the only cure.

6. Sepsis/DIC is a syndrome of anemia, thrombocytopenia, and coagulopathy often occurring in association with a severe, systemic infection. It also occurs in association with malignancies and inflammatory conditions such as pancreatitis.

Patients have rapidly falling hemoglobins and platelet counts, with an elevated partial thromboplastin time. Bleeding and ischemia from clotting may be present. There is a high mortality rate, and improvements occur with treatment of the underlying illness. There may be some benefit in trying to treat severe bleeding (platelet, RBC, and plasma transfusions) or ischemia (heparin) in certain patients, but such treatment is individualized. Treatment of acute promyelocytic leukemia may precipitate DIC, and prophylactic heparin is of benefit.

7. The approach to thrombocytopenia includes a complete history with a careful search for possible causative drugs, infections, or inflammatory conditions, and a physical examination focusing on the spleen and liver. The peripheral blood smear is examined for evidence of clumping, microangiopathic changes, or other abnormalities. If the cause is not certain, then a prompt bone marrow biopsy should be performed. Patients with ITP, TTP, PTP, and other causes of peripheral destruction will have normal or increased numbers of megakaryocytes. A primary marrow disorder may show decreased megakaryocytes or an infiltrative process.

8. Here is a more complete differential for thrombocytopenia:

HELP ME, ITS DIC!

Hemolytic uremic syndrome/TTP
Eclampsia/HEELP/acute fatty liver
Liver disease/portal hypertension
Prosthetic valve

Malignancy/**M**arrow failure
Error (laboratory artifact)

Idiopathic thrombocytopenic purpura
Transfusion (PTP)
Storage diseases/hypersplenism

Drugs (e.g., heparin, antibiotics)
Infections/sepsis
Collagen vascular disease (especially lupus)

THROMBOCYTOSIS

PLATELET CRISIS

Polycythemia vera
Leukemia
Acute hemorrhage
Tumors
Essential thrombocytosis
Lymphoma
Epinephrine
Toxins

Crohn's disease
Rheumatoid arthritis
Infection
Sarcoidosis
Iron deficiency
Splenectomy

Notes

1. Platelets increase in response to systemic processes ("acute phase reactant"). Most cases of thrombocytosis are a reflection of an inflammatory condition. When the platelet count exceeds one million, suspect a primary myeloproliferative disorder such as essential thrombocythemia, polycythemia vera, or leukemia. Bone marrow biopsy is indicated.
2. The four "I"s of thrombocytosis are infection, inflammation, iron deficiency, and increased production.

TRANSFUSION REACTIONS

GOT A BAD UNIT

Graft versus host disease
Overload (iron, volume)
Thrombocytopenia (PTP)

Alloimmunization

Blood pressure instability (anaphylactic)
Acute hemolytic reaction
Delayed hemolytic reaction

Urticaria (allergic cutaneous)
Neutrophilic (febrile)
Infection (HIV, hepatitis, CMV, bacterial sepsis)
Transfusion-associated lung injury (TRALI)

Notes

1. Blood product transfusion is an important and frequently life-saving therapy. Adverse reactions to transfusions are common, however, and thus parsimonious use of this intervention is needed. Transfusion reactions are broadly classified as immune and nonimmune. **Immune causes** include graft versus host disease, post-transfusion thrombocytopenia, alloimmunization, blood pressure instability from anaphylaxis, acute and delayed hemolysis, urticaria, neutrophilic febrile reactions, and TRALI, a neutrophil-induced lung injury. **Nonimmune complications** of transfusion include overload (either acute volume expansion or chronic iron overload) and infections.

2. **Graft versus host disease** (GVHD) is a rare complication of transfusion resulting from transfusion of viable, donor lymphocytes. Transfusion-associated GVHD usually occurs when a patient receives blood from a closely related donor. The donor's lymphocytes have common antigens and are not recognized as foreign by the recipient. These lymphocytes, however, see the recipient as foreign and proliferate, leading to fulminant multiorgan system failure and death.

3. **Overload states**, either volume or iron, are common nonimmune complications of transfusion. In older patients and patients with cardiac disease, the volume of the transfusion may cause pulmonary edema. This complication can

be avoided by slow infusion or administering a diuretic. Iron overload may occur in patients requiring chronic transfusions. This potentially fatal complication can be prevented with chelation therapy.

4. **Thrombocytopenia** is a rare consequence of transfusion. It is usually seen in women with a specific platelet antigen-type, who have had a prior pregnancy. The typical presentation is marked thrombocytopenia occurring several days after a transfusion. Patients spontaneously recover, but steroid therapy or IV immunoglobulin may be of benefit.

5. **Alloimmunization** to blood cell antigens or HLA antigens is common and complicates subsequent transfusions and organ transplantation. Obviously, minimizing exposure to blood products is desirable.

6. **Blood pressure instability** and shock occur in patients with antibodies to IgA. These individuals require IgA-deficient blood products from relatives or rare donor lists.

7. **Acute hemolytic reactions** are rare and often a result of ABO incompatibility or a few other antigens. The cause frequently is clerical error, and the result is rapid intravascular hemolysis. Patients may have flushing, chest and back pain, nausea, diarrhea, dark urine, fever, chills, and shock. Hemoglobinuria, renal failure, DIC, and death may ensue. An important clue to a transfusion reaction is that the hemoglobin does not rise to the expected level after the transfusion. Other helpful laboratory studies include haptoglobin, unconjugated bilirubin, serum and urine free hemoglobins, and a direct Coomb's test. The indirect Coomb's test may not be positive since a great number of antibodies are bound to RBCs.

8. **Delayed hemolytic reactions** are a result of extravascular hemolysis and have a more gradual onset. These reactions most often are caused by antibodies to the Rh system, but others (e.g., Kell, Duffy, Kidd) are common. Malaise, jaundice, and fever occur 5–10 days after transfusion, but more severe complications are rare.

9. **Urticaria** from a cutaneous allergic reaction is a common and benign response to transfusion. It can usually be managed by slowing the infusion and administering antihistamines.

10. **Neutrophilic reactions** usually cause fever and are a result of immune destruction of transfused leukocytes. These reactions are usually mild and treated with antipyretics.

11. **Infections** from transfusion may be caused by viruses, bacteria, or protozoans. The risk of infection is low, but still present. Sterilization is possible for some plasma components, but not for cellular products. Careful donor screening and standard laboratory assays are the most important preventive measures.

12. **Transfusion-associated lung injury** is a rare type of neutrophilic reaction. An allergic pulmonary edema results from lung sequestration of antibody-coated neutrophils. Patients with this more severe reaction have a high titer of antibodies that react with donor leukocytes. With supportive care, most patients have a good recovery.

IV

INFECTIOUS DISEASE

Clinical Symptoms and Signs

FEVER OF UNKNOWN ORIGIN

I GOT THE FEVER*

Inflammatory bowel disease

Granulomatous disease (mycobacteria, fungus, "granulomatous" hepatitis)
Other infections (multiple)
Tumor (especially lymphoma, renal cell carcinoma/hepatoma)

Toxins/medications ("drug fever")
Hypothalamic disease/stroke
Endocarditis

Factitious
Emboli (multiple pulmonary)
Vasculitis
ETOH-induced liver disease
Rheumatologic disease

* differential diagnosis

Notes

1. The classic fever of unknown origin (FUO) was defined as: fevers higher than 38.3°C on several occasions, duration of illness > 3 weeks, and failure to reach a diagnosis after 1 week of inhospital investigation. This has been modified somewhat as many patients are not hospitalized, and special consideration is given to neutropenic, nosocomial, and HIV-associated FUOs.

2. Infections now cause a smaller amount of FUOs because microbiology studies have improved detection. TB; prolonged mononucleosis syndromes with EBV, CMV, and HIV; intra-abdominal abscesses; osteomyelitis; infected prosthetic devices; and endocarditis are considerations. Culture-negative endocarditis is rare, although prior treatment with antibiotics and fastidious organisms ("HACEK"—*Haemophilus aphrophilus*, *Actinobacillus actinomycetemcomitans*, Cardiobacterium, *Eikenella corrodens*, *Kingella kingae*) should be considered.

3. Tumors are less frequent causes due to improved imaging modalities.

4. Factitious fevers are important considerations. Many have occurred in young women in the health professions.

5. In many classic FUOs, there has been an error in the initial work-up. It is imperative to carefully review all previous diagnostic studies (imaging, pathologic specimens, and microbiology) and not simply rely on reports. The patient should be off all medications, if possible, and multiple blood cultures (three to six) should be obtained and be kept for at least 2 weeks to ensure growth of fastidious (i.e., HACEK) organisms. Other specialized culture techniques may be indicated for fungi/atypical mycobacteria, or nutritional variant bacteria. The remainder of the work-up is dictated by the particular case. ESR, febrile agglutinins, and titers for various infectious causes often are obtained, but are probably of low yield. Liver and bone marrow biopsies are routine in FUO work-up, as are imaging studies (usually chest and abdominal CTs). Periodic review and reassessment is critical. After 6 months, a significant portion of FUOs may be undiagnosed (> 20%).

INFECTIONS CAUSING SPLENOMEGALY

THE TREATABLE SPLENIC MASS

Tularemia
Histoplasmosis
EBV (infectious mononucleosis)

Trypanosomiasis, African
Relapsing fever (borelliosis)
Endocarditis
AIDS
Toxicariasis
Acid-fast bacilli (TB and other mycobacteria)
Brucellosis
Leishmaniasis (kala-azar)
Erlichiosis

Salmonella (typhoid fever)
Psittacosis
Lyme disease
Echinococcal cyst
Necrotizing lymphadenitis (Kikuchi's disease)
Infectious hepatitis (viral)
CMV

Malaria
Abscess (bacterial)
Syphilis
Schistosomiasis

Note

Always consider an occult, infectious etiology for splenomegaly since these diseases are likely to respond to appropriate therapy. Listed above is a differential of the numerous infections associated with splenomegaly.

TEMPERATURE-PULSE DISSOCIATION

BAD TEMPS, LO HR

Brucella
Atypical pneumonia (mycoplasma, legionella)
Dengue fever

Tularemia
EBV
Mycobacteria
Psittacosis
Salmonella

Leptospirosis
Orbivirus (Colorado tick fever)

Hepatitis
Rickettsial Illness

Also: yellow fever, "factitious" fever

Note

The clinical finding of a low heart rate with a high temperature may indicate infection with an intracellular pathogen. Older patients with cardiac conduction system disease or on beta-blockers also may have a lower than expected heart rate with fever.

ACUTE MENINGITIS

INFECTS A LOT*

Iatrogenic/post-neurosurgical
***N**eisseria meningitidis*
Fungal
***E**scherichia coli*
Congenital defect/dermal tract
Tuberculous
***S**treptococcus pneumoniae*

Aseptic meningitis (viral)

***L**isteria monocytogenes*
Otitis/mastoiditis/sinusitis
Traumatic bony defect

Also: subarachnoid hemorrhage

* *differential diagnosis*

Notes

Acute meningitis is the abrupt onset of meningeal inflammation, typically associated with infection.

1. Classic symptoms of acute meningitis include fever, headache, stiff neck, and alteration in mental status. In addition, seizures, photophobia, vomiting, and focal neurologic deficits may occur.
2. Work-up of suspected meningitis *must* include examination of CSF:

	Aseptic Meningitis (Viral)	Bacterial Meningitis	Herpes Simplex Encephalitis	TB Meningitis
WBC	10–2000	1000–100,000	0–1000	100–1000
Differential	Early: PMNs Later: lymphs	Mostly PMNs	Mostly lymphs	Early: PMNs Later: lymphs
Glucose	Normal	May be low	Normal	May be low
Protein	Normal	May be high	Normal	May be high

In addition, check CBC and differential for evidence of systemic infection. Check electrolytes, glucose, and BUN/creatinine, and obtain blood cultures. Cranial CT scan is indicated in cases with focal neurologic deficits or evidence of increased intracranial pressure, or if subarachnoid hemorrhage is suspected. Chest and sinus x-rays are helpful in identifying potential sources of infection.

3. Bacterial meningitis is a medical emergency, and diagnosis and treatment must be initiated in a timely fashion. Ideally, CSF should be obtained promptly and antibiotics started as soon as the LP is completed. However, *antibiotics should not be delayed* while awaiting neuroimaging or if there are difficulties in obtaining CSF.

4. Suspected etiologic agents differ with patient's age:

a. Neonates/Infants: *E. coli*, other gram negatives, Group B *streptococcus*, *L. monocytogenes*, rarely *S. pneumoniae*

b. Children: *N. meningitidis*, *S. pneumoniae*. *Haemophilus influenzae* as a cause of childhood meningitis has decreased due to widespread use of *H. influenzae* immunization.

c. Adult: *S. pneumoniae*, *N. meningitidis*. In older populations, *E. coli*, other gram negatives, and *L. monocytogenes* occur with increasing frequency.

5. Other risk factors/clinical findings that may help to determine likely organisms include:

a. Recent neurosurgical procedure—*Staphylococcus aureus*, *S. epidermidis*, anaerobes, gram negatives

b. Brain/epidural abscess, head trauma—anaerobes, gram negatives, *S. pneumoniae*

c. Endocarditis/IV drug use—*S. aureus*

d. Splenectomy, sickle cell disease—*S. pneumoniae*

e. Immunocompromised secondary to chemotherapy, steroids—*S. pneumoniae*, *L. monocytogenes*, fungi, *Mycobacterium tuberculosis*, cytomegalovirus, herpes

f. HIV/AIDS—*Toxoplasma gondii*, *Cryptococcus neoformans*, *M. tuberculosis*, cytomegalovirus, herpes

g. Chronic alcoholism—*S. pneumonaie*, *L. monocytogenes*

h. Congenital defect/dermal tract—*S. aureus*, *S. epidermidis*, *E. coli*, gram negatives

i. Otitis/mastoiditis/sinusitis—*S. pneumoniae*, *H. influenzae*

j. Rash/purpura—*N. meningitidis*

6. Meningismus (stiff neck, nuchal rigidity) is rarely seen in neonates and infants. Likewise, it may not be prominent in elderly, debilitated patients.

7. Subarachnoid hemorrhage may present with alteration in mental status, stiff neck, headache, and even fever.

8. Treatment is directed at likely underlying organisms. Empiric treatment should be initiated as soon as possible and may be changed later as CSF and culture results become available. In neonates, empiric therapy generally consists of ampicillin and gentamicin. In children, cefotaxime or ceftriaxone are used initially; in adults, penicillin G.

AIDS/HUMAN IMMUNODEFICIENCY VIRUS

STOP CATCHING IT*

Salmonella (sepsis, diarrhea)
Thrombocytopenia
Oncologic disease (Kaposi's, lymphoma)
Pneumocystis carinii

Cytomegalovirus, **C**ryptococcosis, **C**andidiasis, **C**ryptosporidium
Avium intracellulare, mycobacterium
Toxoplasmosis
Constitutional symptoms
Herpes simplex/zoster
Iatrogenic
Node enlargement/lymphadenopathy
Guillain Barré syndrome/neuropathy

Isospora
Tuberculosis

Also: dementia

* clinical manifestations/opportunistic infections

Notes

1. Opportunistic infections may be classified according to the organ system(s) involved.

   a. Agents associated with **pneumonia/pneumonitis** include: *Pneumocystis carinii* cytomegalovirus, *Mycobacterium tuberculosis*, herpes simplex.

   b. **Disseminated infections** are seen with *Mycobacterium avium intracellulare*, *Mycobacterium tuberculosis*, cryptococcosis, herpes simplex.

   c. Neurologic infections such as **encephalitis** and **meningitis** are caused by cytomegalovirus, *M. tuberculosis*, cryptococcosis, toxoplasmosis, and direct CNS infection by HIV.

   d. **Ocular infections** usually are associated with cytomegalovirus or toxoplasmosis.

   e. Gastrointestinal (**esophagitis, diarrhea**) manifestations are seen with: cytomegalovirus (esophagitis), candidiasis (esophagitis, oral thrush), herpes simplex (esophagitis), cryptosporidium (diarrhea), isospora (diarrhea), and salmonella (diarrhea).

   f. **Cutaneous infections** are usually due to: herpes simplex and herpes zoster.

2. Oncologic manifestations of AIDS are primarily due to Kaposi's sarcoma and lymphoid malignancies.

3. There are a myriad of neurologic manifestations of AIDS which correlate temporally with the stage of the underlying disease.
   - Asymptomatic
   - Aseptic meningitis, usually early in course
   - Acute demyelinating polyneuropathy (Guillain Barré), usually early
   - Chronic polyneuropathy, later
   - Myelopathy, later
   - Meningitis/encephalitis, opportunistic infection late in course
   - Cerebral neoplasm (primary cerebral lymphoma), late in course
   - Seizures, variable
   - Stroke/ischemia, variable
   - Dementia, late in course

4. Hematologic manifestations of AIDS/HIV
   a. Thrombocytopenia
   b. Anemia
   c. Decreased T4 lymphocyte count

5. Constitutional/systemic symptoms are very common and may be nonspecific, particularly in the early stages of the disease. However, they also may herald the onset of an opportunistic infection, and thus must be taken seriously. These signs and symptoms include fevers, arthralgia, rigors, myalgias, rash, diarrhea, abdominal pain, headache, fatigue, and weight loss.

IMMUNODEFICIENCY STATES

SCANT DISEASE BLOCKS

Skin disease
Complement deficiency
Antibody deficiency
Neutrophil disorders/neutropenia
T-cell abnormalities

Diabetes
Intravenous drug abusers
Splenectomized patients
Elderly
AIDS
Steroids and other immunosuppressive drugs
ETOH abusers

Babies
Liver failure
Organ transplant
Cancer
Kidney failure
Starvation/malnutrition

Notes

1. The "SCANT" part of this mnemonic emphasizes the five major components of the immune system: cutaneous and mucus membrane barriers, complement, antibody, phagocytes, and cell-mediated immunity.
2. Patients with antibody deficiencies have recurrent or chronic sinopulmonary infection, meningitis, and bacteremia, all of which are most commonly caused by pyogenic bacteria.
3. Patients with complement deficiencies are predisposed to pyogenic bacterial infection, and those with terminal complement component deficiencies (C5–C9) may have recurrent Neisseria infections.

4. Abnormalities of T-cells predispose to disseminated viral infections as well as fungi and other opportunistic organisms.

5. Neutropenic patients are predisposed to bacterial and fungal infections.

6. Splenectomized patients are at high risk for severe infections by encapsulated organisms due to *S. pneumoniae*, *H. influenzae*, and *N. meningitidis*. The DF-2 bacillus (*Capnocytophaga canimorsus*) is a fastidious gram-negative organism that may cause fulminant infection after a dog bite. Splenectomized patients also may have more severe illnesses from protozoa such as *Plasmodium malariae* and Babesia.

RHEUMATIC FEVER

JONES*

Joints (polyarthritis)
Overload/opening snap (carditis, valve disease)
Neurologic (chorea)
Erythema marginatum
Subcutaneous nodules

* *major manifestations*

Notes

1. Rheumatic fever is an inflammatory disease that occurs as a delayed sequela to group A streptococcal pharyngeal infection. The diagnosis is made by specific major and minor manifestations of the diseases. The major manifestations of rheumatic fever are summarized by the mnemonic JONES, which refers to the Jones criteria.

2. The **joint involvement** of rheumatic fever is an acute migratory polyarthritis most commonly affecting the large joints of the extremities, but it may affect almost any joint in the body.

3. **Overload/opening snap** refers to the cardiac involvement of rheumatic fever. This is the most important manifestation because it may be fatal in the acute stages or lead to permanent valve damage and long-term cardiac dysfunction.

4. The **neurologic manifestations** of rheumatic fever have been called Sydenham's chorea or St. Vitus' dance, and these names refer to the characteristic

sudden, aimless, irregular movements which may be accompanied by muscle weakness and emotional instability. The chorea is often a delayed manifestation of rheumatic fever.

5. Erythema marginatum is an evanescent pink rash that is characteristic of rheumatic fever. The erythema is transient, migratory, and may be brought on by the application of heat.

6. Subcutaneous nodules are small, pea-sized, painless swellings that occur over bony prominences and tendons.

7. Minor manifestations that can be used in establishing the diagnosis of rheumatic fever include the clinical findings of arthralgia and fever as well as the laboratory findings of an elevated erythrocyte sedimentation rate, an elevated C-reactive protein level, and a prolonged PR interval on the EKG.

8. Evidence supporting an antecedent group A streptococcal infection includes a positive throat culture, a positive rapid streptococcal antigen test, or an elevated or rising streptococcal antibody titer. The diagnosis of rheumatic fever is made by major and minor manifestations, as well as supporting evidence of a group A streptococcal infection. If there is evidence of a preceding group A streptococcal infection and two major manifestations, or one major and two minor manifestations, then there is a high probability that the patient has acute rheumatic fever.

9. Other findings that may be present in a patient with rheumatic fever include abdominal pain, tachycardia, and epistaxis, but these findings are nonspecific and of minor diagnostic value.

SEXUALLY TRANSMITTED DISEASES

NO WRAP, U GETS CLAP*

NOngonococcal urethritis

Warts, genital
Reiter's syndrome
AIDS
Proctitis, infectious

Ulcerative genital lesions (herpes simplex)

Gonorrhea
Epididymitis
Trichomonas
Syphilis

Cytomegalovirus, **C**ervical cancer
Lice
Arthritis
Pelvic inflammatory disease

* *differential diagnosis*

Notes

1. Clinical symptoms that bring sexually transmitted diseases (STDs) to a physician's attention include genital discharge, pain/discomfort, or visible lesions. Many patients with STDs are asymptomatic and do not seek medical care.
2. Proper management of a patient with an STD must include identification and treatment of the infected partner.
3. It is helpful to classify STDs into common clinical presentations or syndromes:

a. Urethritis (males)	f. Proctitis/lower GI infections
b. Epididymitis	g. Acute arthritis
c. Urethritis/cystitis (females)	h. Warts
d. Vulvovaginitis	i. Pelvic inflammatory disease (females)
e. Ulcerative lesions	

4. Urethritis typically presents as a urethral discharge and/or dysuria in a sexually active male. The most likely agents are *N. gonorrheae, Chlamydia trachomatis, Ureaplasma urealyticum,* and herpes simplex virus. Alternate diagnoses to be considered include bacterial cystitis or prostatitis.
5. Epididymitis may present as unilateral testicular pain. The differential diagnosis includes testicular torsion, trauma, testicular cancer, or infection. As in urethritis, *N. gonorrheae* and *C. trachomatis* are the predominant agents. Gram negatives may cause epididymitis in older men or after urinary tract procedures.
6. Lower genitourinary infections in females present with vaginal discharge, dysuria, painful intercourse, and/or genital discomfort. Urethritis/cystitis generally causes dysuria and is due to *N. gonorrheae, C. trachomatis,* or bacterial cystitis. Vulvovaginitis typically manifests with vaginal discharge, vaginal pain/discomfort, and "dysuria" due to contact of urine with inflamed labia. Primary etiologic agents are yeasts (*Candida albicans*), *Trichomonas vaginalis,* and bacteria (*Gardnerella vaginalis,* mycoplasma, etc.).
7. Genital ulcers are caused by the following organisms:
    a. *Treponema pallidum* (syphilis)

     i. Lesion (chancre): ulcerated, painless, firm, indurated papule. Incubation 10–90 days.

     ii. Adenopathy: firm, discrete, movable, painless, occurring 1 week after chancre.

  b. *Herpes genitalis*

     i. Lesion: multiple, painful, erythematous vesicles. Incubation 2–7 days.

     ii. Adenopathy: tender, soft; not prominent with recurrent lesions.

  c. *Haemophilus ducreyi* (chancroid)

     i. Lesion: soft, not indurated, very painful vesicle/papule to ulcer. Incubation 3–5 days.

     ii. Adenopathy: painful, unilateral, suppurative, occurring 1 week after primary.

  d. *Chlamydia trachomatis* (lymphogranuloma venereum)

     i. Lesion: painless, often unnoticed papule/ulcer. Incubation 5–21 days.

     ii. Adenopathy: tender, bilateral (33%), matted, suppurative, occurring 5–21 days after.

  e. *Calymmatobacterium granulomatis* (granuloma inguinale)

     i. Lesion: painless, irregular, thickened papule/ulcer. Incubation 9–50 days.

     ii. Adenopathy: none. May develop groin abscesses, however.

8. Acute arthritis is most commonly caused by *N. gonorrheae* in young adults. Reiter's syndrome is second. Differential diagnosis includes other infectious arthritides (*meningococcus, Yersinia,* syphilis), crystal-induced arthritis, RA, SLE, and sarcoid. See the differential for acute monoarthritis in the Rheumatology chapter for more information.

9. Genital warts (condyloma acuminata) are caused by human papillomavirus and are associated with cervical dysplasia. The differential diagnosis of warts includes condyloma lata (secondary syphilis) and molluscum contagiosum.

10. Pelvic inflammatory disease is typically caused by *N. gonorrheae* or *C. trachomatis.* Symptomatology includes lower abdominal/pelvic pain, often during menses, and sometimes cervical discharge, pelvic mass, and/or leukocytosis.

V

Cardiology

Clinical Symptoms and Signs

Syncope

ACLS

Anxiety
Cardiovascular causes
Loss of volume/orthostasis
Seizure/neurologic causes

Also: see "Loss of consciousness" in the Neurology chapter.

Notes

1. Syncope is a generalized weakness of muscles with loss of postural tone, inability to stand upright, and a loss of consciousness. There are many causes of syncope, and it must be differentiated from feelings of dizziness or faintness as well as seizures. Since patients often present with a loss of consciousness without a clear history of antecedent events, we include seizures in the differential diagnosis of syncope even though strictly speaking they do not cause syncope.

2. The mnemonic ACLS gives a simple grouping for the causes of apparent syncope. **Anxiety** or emotional stress may cause a loss of consciousness and subsequent syncope. **Cardiovascular causes** include congestive heart failure, valvular heart disease, impaired venous return, and arrhythmias. **Loss of volume** causes hypotension and subsequent orthostasis. Examples include blood loss from gastrointestinal hemorrhage, dehydration, and Addison's disease. **Seizures**

or neurologic disorders also can cause a loss of consciousness. Again, the differentiation between seizures and the true causes of syncope is a critical aspect of the evaluation. A more comprehensive and mechanistic approach to the problem of syncope is summarized by the following mnemonic:

VASOVAGALS

Volume loss
Anxiety attack
Seizure/CVA
Obstruction of venous return (micturition, Valsalva, cough, myxoma)
Vasodepressor/**V**asoconstrictor defect
Arrhythmia
Glucose drop
Aortic dissection
Low cardiac output
Shy-Drager/**S**ympathetic dysfunction

3. VASOVAGALS outlines the causes of syncope according to the physiologic mechanisms. **Volume loss, anxiety attacks, and seizures/CVA** are again important considerations. **Obstruction of venous return** may occur with micturition, Valsalva maneuvers, cough, or, rarely, a ball-valve effect of an atrial myxoma.

Vasodepressor/vasoconstrictor defects may precipitate neurocardiogenic syncope. Syncope in this setting typically occurs when there is a diminished venous return to the heart upon standing. This diminished venous return leads to a reduction in stroke volume and a reflex increase in sympathetic activity. In susceptible individuals, the increased sympathetic activity causes a complex interaction between the heart and the autonomic nervous system. The net result is inappropriate peripheral vasodilation and bradycardia, which precipitate hypotension and syncope. The diagnosis is made by tilt-table testing, often using isoproterenol infusion. Neurocardiogenic syncope often responds well to beta-blocker therapy.

Cardiac **arrhythmias**, either tachyarrhythmias or bradyarrhythmias, are important in potentially life-threatening causes of syncope. Arrhythmias often indicate the presence of ischemic or mechanical cardiac disease.

4. A blood **glucose drop** also can cause faintness and a syncopal event. In severe cases, low glucose levels may induce seizures. Insulin-dependent diabetics and elderly patients on oral hypoglycemic agents are at risk.

5. **Aortic dissection** is a less common cause of syncope, and the diagnosis is often unsuspected. Aortic dissection can be rapidly fatal, and the symptoms may be relatively nonspecific. The dissection may cause a loss of blood volume or pericardial tamponade and resulting syncope. A **low cardiac output** may be

secondary to congestive heart failure; valvular heart disease, especially aortic stenosis; massive pulmonary embolism; or cardiac tamponade. A high level of suspicion and prompt diagnosis may be lifesaving.

6. Finally, **Shy-Drager/sympathetic dysfunction** refers to peripheral autonomic dysfunction that causes a vasoconstrictor defect. Shy-Drager syndrome is an idiopathic autonomic disorder. Surgical sympathectomy or pharmacologic sympathectomy due to antihypertensive medications can cause inadequate vasoconstriction when assuming an upright posture. Diabetic neuropathy or infiltrative diseases such as amyloidosis are common causes. Cerebral hypoperfusion results with a subsequent syncopal episode.

7. *Differentiating syncope from seizure is critical.* Seizure patients more often have no memory of the events preceding the event and demonstrate post-event (postictal) confusion. Also, severe injury from falling, tongue biting, and incontinence are indicative of a seizure.

8. A comprehensive list of the individual entities causing syncope is summarized by the mnemonic THIS MADE ME DAMN VAGAL.

THIS MADE ME DAMN VAGAL

Tamponade
Hypertensive crisis
Intracranial hemorrhage/CVA
Seizure

Myocardial infarction
Aortic dissection
Drugs
Emotion/anxiety attack

Micturition/tussive
Embolus (PE)

Dysrhythmia
Addison's
Migraine (basilar)
Neurocardiogenic

Volume loss
Aortic stenosis/obstruction
Glucose drop
Autonomic dysfunction
Low cardiac output (CHF)

ARRHYTHMIA

AICD ME?

Adrenergic stimuli
Ischemia
Conduction system disease
Drugs

Mechanical stimuli (e.g., stretch, PA catheter)
Electrolytes

Notes

1. Cardiac arrhythmia can be subdivided into **tachyarrhythmias** or **brady-arrhythmias**. Although the electrophysiologic mechanisms of arrhythmia are complex, a few basic etiologies should be considered in every patient with an arrhythmia. These mechanisms are summarized by the mnemonic "AICD ME?" The mnemonic also asks the clinical question of whether an automatic implantable cardiac defibrillator (AICD) is indicated. This form of therapy is becoming increasingly common, particularly for patients with ventricular arrhythmias and congestive heart failure.

2. **Adrenergic stimuli** may precipitate cardiac tachyarrhythmias. Examples include excessive caffeine intake, beta-adrenergic agonists, and pheochromocytoma. Cardiac **ischemia** also is an important consideration in arrhythmia. Ischemic damage to the conduction system may set up the substrate for arrhythmia, or resultant congestive heart failure may cause myocardial stretch and also precipitate arrhythmias. **Conduction system disease** can be congenital or secondary to ischemia or mechanical stimuli. **Drugs** are a common precipitant of cardiac arrhythmias. In addition to **adrenergic stimuli**, agents such as cisapride and terfenadine in combination with macrolide antibiotics have been implicated as etiologies of cardiac arrhythmia. Many agents used to treat cardiac arrhythmias may have proarrhythmic effects. **Mechanical stimuli** can precipitate

cardiac arrhythmia. Finally, **electrolyte** abnormalities, especially perturbations in potassium, magnesium, and calcium, are important considerations in a patient with cardiac arrhythmias.

ATRIAL FIBRILLATION

I HAVE A FIB

Ischemia

Hyperthyroidism
Acute pericarditis
Valvular heart disease (especially mitral stenosis)
Embolus (PE)

Atrial septal defect
Failure (CHF)
Infection
Booze

Notes

1. Atrial fibrillation is a common arrhythmia that can be intermittent (paroxysmal) or persistent. It is characterized by disorganized atrial activity with an "irregularly irregular" ventricular response. The major morbidities of atrial fibrillation are:

　a. Tachycardia that may precipitate hypotension, syncope, pulmonary edema, or angina

　b. Loss of "atrial kick" that facilitates left ventricular filling and output

　c. Systemic emboli most often causing stroke. Most patients with chronic atrial fibrillation should be considered for warfarin anticoagulation (target INR of 2.0–3.0) to reduce the risk of cerebrovascular accident.

2. After initial rate control of symptomatic atrial fibrillation, search for an etiology. Most often, underlying cardiopulmonary disease such as **pericarditis, valvular heart disease, atrial septal defect**, or **failure** (left sided or right sided) is present. Myocardial infarction is a rare cause of *isolated* atrial fibrillation, but patients with ischemic heart disease may develop atrial fibrillation over time.

3. Investigate other primary causes or factors that may unmask atrial fibrillation in a susceptible individual. Atrial fibrillation may be the first sign of **hyperthyroidism** or **pulmonary embolism.** Systemic disorders such as **infection** also can precipitate atrial fibrillation. **Booze** ingestion may precipitate a variety of arrhythmias, including atrial fibrillation. The so-called holiday heart typically occurs after a binge drinking episode on a weekend.

4. Rarely, atrial fibrillation occurs without associated heart disease or the above-listed precipitants. This "lone" atrial fibrillation generally has a good long-term prognosis and may be a manifestation of underlying tachycardia-bradycardia syndrome.

CONGESTIVE HEART FAILURE

ISCHEMIA? PA CATHS

Low output
Ischemia
Subacute bacterial endocarditis
Cardiomyopathy
Hypertension
Effusion/tamponade
Mitral valve disease
Infectious myocarditis
Aortic valve disease

High output
Paget/myeloma
A-V fistula

Cardiac shunt
Anemia
Thiamine deficiency (beri-beri)
Hyperthyroidism
Sepsis

Notes

1. Congestive heart failure (CHF) is a **clinical diagnosis**. If a careful physical examination reveals the findings of CHF (edema, jugular venous distention, a right or left-sided heave, an auscultatory S3 or S4, rales, pleural effusions), then regardless of other diagnostic testing results, the patient is in clinical CHF. The importance of the physical examination findings cannot be over-emphasized: there are many forms of CHF in which cardiac function may appear normal on imaging studies. Once a careful clinical examination is done, and the patient has been determined to be clinically in CHF, clinical imaging studies such as an echocardiogram may be used to confirm the diagnosis and to elucidate the etiology.

2. The mnemonic "ISCHEMIA? PA CATHS" divides congestive heart failure into two main types: those associated with low cardiac output, and those associated with high cardiac output. When a careful examination reveals the clinical features of CHF, but the echocardiogram shows a normal ejection fraction, consider one of three possibilities:
   a. The echocardiogram is suboptimal.
   b. High-output CHF is present.
   c. A diastolic, restrictive or constrictive defect is present.

3. Low-output states are the most common causes of CHF. **Ischemia** with subsequent left ventricular dysfunction is the most common cause of CHF and potentially reversible. **Subacute bacterial endocarditis** may cause tachycardia and vasodilation, stressing the heart. It also can cause valvular injury and subsequent stenosis or regurgitation. Idiopathic **cardiomyopathy**, also called dilated cardiomyopathy, causes CHF in the absence of coronary artery disease. Long-standing **hypertension** may cause cardiac dysfunction in a low-output state. Hypertension also can cause a restrictive cardiomyopathy. Pericardial **effusion** or **tamponade** may cause symptoms of CHF, and should be detected by echocardiography. **Mitral** and **aortic** valvular diseases are less common today, but still important causes of CHF. Again, echocardiography is useful to rule out these entities. Finally, **infection**, usually viral, may cause myocarditis and a subsequent dilated cardiomyopathy.

4. High-output failure is less common than the low-output states. "PA CATHS" summarizes the causes of high-output failure. It also indicates the most important test to perform when a patient is in CHF, but the echocardiogram suggests normal systolic function: pulmonary artery catheterization. The abnormal physiology of the high-output state may be secondary to a systemic shunt, as occurs with **Paget's disease** and **multiple myeloma**. In these diseases there are bony, intramedullary shunts. There is increased blood flow through these shunts without tissue oxygen delivery. The result is an increase in SVO_2 and increased demand on the heart to maintain a higher cardiac output to meet the oxygen demands of the other tissues in the body. A large **arteriovenous fistula** or **cardiac shunt** may have the same effect. Severe **anemia** reduces the oxygen carrying capacity of the blood, forcing the heart to maintain a higher cardiac output. **Thiamine deficiency** causes diffuse vasodilatation which in turn leads to an increased volume of circulation that the

heart must maintain. A characteristic hyperdynamic circulation is seen. **Hyperthyroidism**, with its heightened metabolic demands, also can cause a high-output state. **Sepsis** leads to a high-output state with systemic vasodilatation. Again, in these conditions the heart is under stress, and failure may ensue. Sepsis also may have a direct cardiac depressant effect, and this can exacerbate circulatory failure. In restrictive diseases, the cardiac output may be normal or high.

5. In a patient with known CHF, decompensation may occur, leading to an **edematous** state with pedal edema, or "**edema toes**." The following mnemonic summarizes the important considerations in decompensated CHF. All of these entities should be considered when determining the cause of CHF exacerbation.

EDEMA TOES

Embolus
Dysrhythmia
Eclampsia/pregnancy
Myocardial infarction
Anemia

Thyroid disease
Overexertion/excessive fluid or salt
Elevated blood pressure
Sepsis/infection

6. Although most CHF is due to systolic dysfunction, certain conditions may impede the heart's ability to relax. This "diastolic dysfunction" impedes cardiac filling and leads to the clinical state of CHF. The distinguishing feature is a normal left ventricular ejection fraction on an echocardiogram or other imaging test. Remember that the left ventricular ejection fraction is a measure of *systolic* function, but does not assess the heart's diastolic function.

HYPOTENSION

BP DECLINED

Blood loss
Poor PO intake

Diarrhea/**D**ehydration
Endocrine (e.g., Addison's)
Cardiac disease
Liver failure
Infection/sepsis
Neuropathy (autonomic)
Embolus (pulmonary)
Drugs

Notes

1. This differential shares many of the features of syncope.
2. Addison's disease may look very much like sepsis with fever, altered mental status, and refractory hypotension. It is rapidly improved (minutes) with intravenous glucocorticoids.

PERICARDITIS

PR DIP, ST UP

Post-pericardiotomy
Rheumatic fever

Drugs
Infection (TB, viral, pyogenic)
Pulmonary embolus

SLE
Thyroid disease

Uremia
Post-MI (acute, Dressler)

Notes

1. Pericarditis is a syndrome caused by inflammation of the pericardium. The results of this inflammation include chest pain, a pericardial friction rub, pericardial effusion, and characteristic EKG changes.
2. Chest pain (often severe) is a common symptom of acute pericarditis. It may be absent in more subacute disease, such as tuberculosis or myxedema. Characteristically, the pain is relieved by sitting up and leaning forward. Swallowing may exacerbate the pain.
3. Pericardial friction rub is the most important physical sign. It is a high-pitched, scratching sound and may have three components corresponding to the cardiac cycle.
4. "PR DIP, ST UP" describes the characteristic EKG changes in paricarditis: depression of the PR intervals and widespread elevation of ST segments. T wave inversion also may be seen. Differentiation of these EKG changes from those of acute myocardial ischemia is important.
5. Here is a mnemonic for the differential diagnosis of pericarditis:

IT CAUSED PERICARDITIS

Infection (viral, bacterial, mycobacterial, fungal, parasitic)
Tumor (primary, metastatic)

Collagen-vascular diseases (e.g., SLE, RA, scleroderma)
Acute MI
Uremia
Sarcoidosis
Embolus
Dressler's

Post-pericardiotomy
External trauma
Rheumatic fever
Inherited (familial, FMF)
Cholesterol/**C**hylopericardium
Atrial septal defect
Ruptured aortic aneurysm
Drugs (procainamide, hydralazine, and others)
Idiopathic

Thyroid disease (myxedema)
Irradiation
Severe, chronic anemia

6. Inflammation of the pericardium may be secondary to an **infection**, usually viral, but bacterial, mycobacterial, and other etiologies are possible. Inflammation also may occur as a result of direct injury to the pericardium, such as **post-cardiac surgery**, or from **chest trauma**. Adjacent inflammation of the lung, as occurs with pulmonary **embolism**, or the heart, as occurs with **acute myocardial infarction**, also can cause pericarditis. Myocardial infarction may cause an acute pericardial effusion or a later, autoimmune phenomenon called **Dressler's** syndrome. Dressler's syndrome also can occur after cardiac surgery. Other **collagen-vascular diseases** such as rheumatoid arthritis or systemic lupus erythematosus commonly cause pericardial disease. Pericarditis is also one of the cardiac manifestations of **rheumatic fever**. Systemic illnesses such as **uremia** and **hypothyroidism** can cause pericardial inflammation and effusion. Finally, certain **drugs** may cause pericardial disease and/or effusion including hydralazine, procainamide, and minoxidil.

RESTRICTIVE CARDIAC DISEASE

A STIFFER CHF

Amyloid

Sarcoidosis
Tumor infiltration
Idiopathic
Fibrosis (endomyocardial)
Fabry's
Eosinophilic
Radiation

Constrictive pericarditis
Hypertension/**H**ypertrophy
Fe overload (hemochromotosis)

Note

This mnemonic lists those infiltrative and fibrotic diseases that lead to diastolic dysfunction. Also included in this list is the entity of **constrictive pericarditis**, which may be difficult to distinguish from restrictive disease even after echocardiography and pulmonary artery catheterization. The differentiation of constrictive pericarditis from restrictive disease is critical, because constrictive pericarditis is surgically correctable.

VI

ENDOCRINOLOGY

General Considerations

Endocrine disorders present in myriad ways and are a category in the MEDI-CINE DOC mnemonic. Critical to the understanding of these disorders is the concept of a stimulatory signal (**"trophic" hormone**) from a remote source and a target gland that produces the **"effector" hormone**. Feedback from the target organ or from a metabolic product further downstream is often responsible for the subsequent inhibition of the trophic hormone. Because of this regulatory system, endocrine disorders may result from dysfunction of the stimulatory or the effector organs. When considering endocrine disease, think about the consequences of **hyper-** and **hypo-function** of each effector gland and its stimulatory gland.

Note that standard endocrinologic testing is best done in an out-patient setting when the patient is in a stable state of health. Acute illnesses in hospitalized patients can unpredictably alter hormonal testing and make test interpretation unreliable.

Pituitary/Hypothalamus

The pituitary is the master, or **"TOP GLAND,"** (see next page) because it produces six major hormones (TSH, prolactin, growth hormone, the gonadotropins LH and FSH, and ACTH), and stores two others (ADH and oxytocin). The pituitary-hypothalamic axis is a tripartite system consisting of the anterior pituitary ("TOP GLA"), the posterior pituitary or neurohypophysis ("N") and the hypothalamus ("D"). The posterior pituitary is essentially an extension of an area of the hypothalamus. The **optic chiasm** lies anterior and superior to the pituitary gland and is compressed by anterior pituitary neoplasms causing visual field defects. Visual symptoms may be the first sign of a pituitary tumor. The anterior pituitary is a major producer of endogenous **opiates**, including endorphins, enkephalins, and dynorphins.

    TSH
    Optic chiasm/Opioids
    Prolactin

Growth hormone
LH/FSH
ACTH
Neurohypophysis (ADH, oxytocin)
Dopamine/hypothalamic releasing factors

Anterior Pituitary: Hypo- and Hyper-Function

TSH. Symptoms of hypofunction are those of hypothyroidism, including fatigue, lethargy, constipation, cold intolerance, muscle cramps, carpal tunnel syndrome, menorrhagia, edema, weight loss, slowing of intellectual function, dry skin and hair, deepening of the voice, and coma. Signs of hyperfunction are those of hyperthyroidism (see Hyperthyroidism section).

Optic chiasm. Although not a hormone-secreting entity, anterior pituitary tumors impinge upon this structure and cause visual field disturbances.

Prolactin. High levels of prolactin may cause hypogonadism and galactorrhea, while low levels are characterized by the inability to lactate.

Growth hormone. Excess growth hormone causes acromegaly, a syndrome that may include fatigue, increased sweating, heat intolerance, enlarging hands and feet, coarsening of facial features, headache, vision loss, macroglossia, CHF, impotence, kidney stones, hypersomnolence, and obstructive sleep apnea.

LH and FSH. Deficiency of the gonadotropins results in hypogonadism and infertility. Gonadotropin excess is usually diagnosed in men with decreased libido, and may be misdiagnosed as primary hypogonadism if a pituitary tumor is not suspected.

ACTH. ACTH excess results in Cushing's syndrome, characterized by muscle weakness, hypertension, amenorrhea, glucose intolerance, osteoporosis, striae, and central distribution of fat. ACTH deficiency causes secondary adrenal insufficiency (see Adrenal Insufficiency section).

Neurohypophysis (Posterior Pituitary): Hypo- and Hyper-Function

ADH. ADH excess is reviewed in the SIADH section. Loss of ADH causes diabetes insipidus (see Hypernatremia section in the Nephrology chapter).

Oxytocin. Oxytocin stimulates uterine contraction and contraction of myoepithelial cells of the breast, causing milk ejection. Oxytocin has an ADH-like effect, which may be clinically significant when it is given in large doses for obstetrical uses. It also has a vasodilatory effect, which may cause hypotension and cardiovascular compromise, particularly in patients with heart disease and when anesthetics are coadministered.

Hypothalamus: Hypo- and Hyper-Function

Dopamine (prolactin-releasing factor) and the hypophysiotropic hormones (TRH, CRH, LHRH, GHRH, and GIH [somatostatin]) are produced by the hypothalamus and regulate prolactin release, thyroid function, the adrenal axis, gonadotropins, and growth hormone release. Injury to the hypothalamus or pituitary stalk results in a reduction in levels of GH, LH, FSH, TSH, and ACTH, with a rise in prolactin, which is normally inhibited by tonic release of dopamine. Arginine vasopressin and oxytocin levels fall if the neurohypophysis is injured.

Clinical Symptoms and Signs

AMENORRHEA

WHAT SEX?*

Weight loss
Hypothalamic (pituitary dysfunction)
Anatomic anomalies of the vagina and uterus
Testicular feminization

Stress (systemic illness)
Exercise
XO (Turner's)

Also: Gonadal dysgenesis, Kallman's syndrome, physiologic delay

* primary amenorrhea

PERIOD GAP*

Polycystic ovary disease/insulin resistance
Endometrial failure (Asherman's)
Resistant ovary syndrome
Illness (severe systemic disease)
Ovarian failure (autoimmune, early menopause)
Dieting/exercise

Gravid
Adrenal dysfunction (congenital adrenal hyperplasia,
   Addison's)
Pituitary disease

* *secondary amenorrhea*

Notes

1. Amenorrhea is divided into primary (no initiation of menses) and secondary (cessation of established menses) categories.
2. Pregnancy must be ruled out first in any patient with amenorrhea. Further evaluation is generally undertaken in the following instances:
   a. No menses have occurred by age 14, and development of secondary sex characteristics is absent or retarded.
   b. No menses have occurred by age 16.
   c. A woman with established menses has no bleeding for three cycles or 6 months.
3. The basic categories of problems are outflow problems (anatomic block), ovarian disorders, anterior pituitary disorders, and CNS disorder (hypothalamus).
4. Evaluation *after pregnancy is ruled out* includes a history and physical exam, with a clinical assessment of estrogen status. On pelvic examination, normal estrogen-stimulated vaginal mucosa is moist and rugated. Normal cervical mucus stretches and demonstrates ferning when placed on a slide.
5. If clinical examination is normal, a TSH and prolactin are obtained, and the patient is given a progestational challenge to check for withdrawal menses. If withdrawal bleeding occurs and prolactin and TSH are normal, then the diagnosis is anovulatory bleeding (polycystic ovarian disease). If no withdrawal bleeding occurs, then evaluation depends upon the prolactin level. If prolactin is elevated and/or galactorrhea is present, then pituitary imaging is indicated. If prolactin is low or normal, then LH and FSH should be measured. If LH and FSH are elevated, then the diagnosis is ovarian failure. If gonadotropins are low or normal, then the diagnosis is a hypothalamic-pituitary disorder or an anatomic uterine defect (e.g., Asherman's). Cyclic estrogen and progesterone should cause menstruation if the uterus is normal.

GYNECOMASTIA

TEST ME

Testosterone deficiency
Estrogen excess
Senility
Teenagers/infants

Medications
Etiology unknown

Notes

1. Gynecomastia does not indicate absolute hormone levels, but rather a change in the ratio of male to female sex hormones. Gynecomastia may be indicative of underlying endocrinopathy or may be the result of obesity or a normal physiologic phenomenon (newborn, adolescence, aging).

2. Causes of gynecomastia can be classified as either pathologic or physiologic. Pathologic causes may be divided into those which lead to a **decrease in testosterone** level, an **increase in estrogen** level, or are secondary to the effect of a **medication**. A decreased testosterone level may be the result of a congenital disorder or testicular failure secondary to renal failure, trauma, or orchitis. Increased estrogen effect may be secondary to a primary increase in estrogen, such as occurs with tumors of the testes, true hermaphrodites, or hCG-producing tumors. An increased estrogen effect also may be seen when there is increased substrate available for extra-glandular aromatase, such as occurs in adrenal disease, liver disease, malnutrition, or hyperthyroidism. A primary increase in extraglandular aromatase also can lead to increased estrogen effect. Physiologic causes are those changes that occur during the normal human lifetime such as in **newborns, teenagers**, and the **elderly**. Most cases are idiopathic (**etiology unknown**). A definitive diagnosis can be reached in less than one-half of patients.

3. Physical examination should include testicular examination. If testes are small, obtain a karyotype. If testes are asymmetric, a tumor may be present.

4. Initial laboratory tests include liver and renal function tests. Endocrine evaluation includes measurements of serum androstenedione or 24-hour urinary 17-ketosteroids, plasma estradiol, hCG, LH, and testosterone.

5. Drugs may cause gynecomastia by **pro-estrogenic or anti-testosterone mechanisms**. They may act directly as estrogens, enhance estrogen secretion,

inhibit testosterone action or synthesis, or act by an unknown mechanism. A careful drug history is essential. Drugs that cause gynecomastia include estrogens, ketoconazole, metronidazole, various chemotherapeutic agents, spironolactone, cimetidine, flutamide, isoniazid, methyl dopa, tricyclic antidepressants, omeprazole, ACE inhibitors, calcium-channel blockers, marijuana, and heroin.

6. Men with Klinefelter's syndrome have a high incidence of breast cancer. Screening mammography is essential.

7. Here is a more comprehensive list of the causes of gynecomastia:

NUDE TESTAMENT

Newborn/teenager
Uremia/renal failure
Drugs
Estrogens

Testosterone inhibitors
Elderly
Starvation/nutritional deficiency
Testicular failure
Adrenal disease
Morbid obesity (high aromatase)
End-stage liver disease
Neoplasm (testicular or other HCG-producing tumor)
Thyroid disease

HIRSUTISM

PCOD HAIRS

Prolactinoma
Congenital adrenal hyperplasia
Ovarian tumors (arrhenoblastoma, hilus cell tumor)
Drugs

Hilus cell hyperplasia
Adrenal tumors
Idiopathic (familial)
Resistance to insulin (syndrome X, polycystic ovary
   disease)
Steroids (exogenous, Cushing's)

Also: idiopathic (familial)

Notes

1. Hirsutism is defined as **male-pattern** hair growth in women, in contrast to hypertrichosis, which is excessive hair growth in a normal body distribution. Hirsutism is due to a hormonal imbalance (i.e., excessive androgen production), while hypertrichosis results from stimulation of existing hair, often by medications (e.g., cyclosporin or minoxidil). There is considerable variability in hair growth in normal men and women; thus abnormal hair growth is difficult to define.

2. The clinical scenario dictates the diagnostic evaluation of hirsutism. Polycystic ovary disease ("PCOD") is one of the most common causes of pathologic hirsutism and is subacute in onset. Rapid onset and frank virilization are characteristic of malignancies and mandate complete evaluation.

3. The history should focus on drug ingestion, family history, and menstrual history. Physical examination signs of virilization include deepening of voice (laryngeal enlargement), temporal balding, clitoromegaly, male escutcheon, and increased muscle mass. Signs of Cushing's syndrome (stria, moon face, truncal obesity, and "buffalo hump") should be sought.

4. Obtain plasma testosterone, prolactin, and DHEAS levels, possibly followed by adrenal and ovarian imaging.

5. Most patients on steroid therapy do not have hirsutism, because steroids suppress adrenal androgen production. Androgen production is stimulated by ACTH, so only conditions featuring excessive ACTH secretion typically cause hirsutism.

6. Drugs (and polycystic ovary disease or Stein-Leventhal syndrome) are the most common causes of nonfamilial hirsutism. True drug-induced hirsutism (in contrast to hypertrichosis) results from a direct androgenic effect or stimulation of androgen secretion.

7. Congenital adrenal hyperplasia (late 21-hydroxylase deficiency) may be clinically indistinguishable from PCOD. Patients with this disorder have a defect in cortisol synthesis leading to elevated ACTH levels, which in turn cause excessive androgen production. Elevated DHEAS and dexamethesone-suppressible hyperandrogenism are strong supports for this diagnosis.

8. Patients with Cushing's syndrome may not always have hirsutism. Glucocorticoids suppress adrenal androgen production. ACTH stimulates androgen production.

ADRENAL INSUFFICIENCY

LACKS ADRENAL*

Low sodium
Acidosis
Calcium elevation
K+ elevation
Skin hyperpigmentation

Altered mental status
Depression
Refractory hypotension
Eosinophilia
Nausea/abdominal pain/anorexia
Asthenia
Loss of weight

* *characteristics of adrenal insufficiency*

Notes

1. Primary adrenocortical deficiency is rare, but secondary (due to steroid therapy) is relatively common. Adrenal insufficiency may be unmasked by stress due to, for example, systemic illness or infection.
2. **Causes of adrenal insufficiency** include anatomic destruction of the adrenals (autoimmune destruction, surgical removal, infection, hemorrhage, or metastatic invasion), metabolic failure (congenital adrenal hyperplasia or enzyme inhibitors such as metapyrone or ketoconazole), ACTH-blocking antibodies, suppression of the hypothalamic-pituitary axis due to steroid therapy, and hypopituitarism secondary to hypothalamic-pituitary disease.
3. Primary adrenal insufficiency may be part of a polyglandular autoimmune syndrome. Associated conditions include lymphocytic thyroiditis, premature ovarian failure, diabetes, and hyperthyroidism. Additional disorders include pernicious anemia, vitiligo, alopecia, sprue, and myasthenia gravis.

4. **Laboratory diagnosis** of adrenal insufficiency requires ACTH stimulation testing to assess adrenal reserve capacity for steroid production. Serum and urinary steroid levels may be in the normal range in mild adrenal insufficiency, and therefore are not reliable for diagnosis. Basal levels of cortisol and aldosterone may be subnormal, but definitive diagnosis is obtained when they fail to increase after ACTH stimulation.

5. Consider adrenal insufficiency in any patient on steroid therapy, since duration of therapy cannot reliably predict which patients will have suppression of the adrenal axis. Patients on steroid therapy who have significant intercurrent illness should be given stress-dose steroids empirically while acutely ill.

6. Solumedrol and prednisone interfere with the ACTH stimulation test. Hydrocortisone therapy makes interpretation of the test difficult, as well. In a patient with suspected adrenal insufficiency, dexamethasone may be given acutely, as it will not interfere with the ACTH stimulation test. Both solumedrol and prednisone are ultimately converted to prednisolone, which directly interferes with the cortisol assay. Hydrocortisone also directly interferes with the cortisol assay. Dexamethasone does not interfere, but if it is given over several days it can suppress the adrenal axis. Dexamethasone also has very little mineralocorticoid effect and may not improve hypotension as dramatically as hydrocortisone.

7. In critically ill patients, interpretation of the ACTH stimulation test is difficult, and free cortisol levels vary greatly. At this time, there is no convincing evidence that steroid supplementation is beneficial in these patients in the absence of clearly demonstrable adrenal insufficiency.

CARCINOID TUMORS

5-HIAAS

Heart
Intestine
Airway
Asthma
Skin

Notes

1. Carcinoid tumors are thought to arise from neuroendocrine cells. They synthesize a variety of hormones and biogenic amines; the most prominent of these

substances is **serotonin**. Serotonin is metabolized in the body to 5-hydroxyin-doleacetic acid (5-HIAA), which is then excreted in the urine. Serotonin is the major mediator responsible for cardinal manifestations of the carcinoid syndrome, and these five manifestations are conveniently outlined by the mnemonic "5-HIAAS."

2. Carcinoid tumors can be found in a number of locations. The lungs, bronchi, and trachea are the most common sites for a carcinoid. Other sites include the stomach, duodenum, jejunum, ileum, appendix, cecum, colon, and rectum. In general, the carcinoid syndrome, with all its systemic manifestations, is seen in patients with metastatic disease to the liver. This is thought to occur because the enteropathic circulation normally metabolizes the products of the carcinoid tumor, thus preventing systemic symptoms. Once hepatic metastases are present, the products produced by the carcinoid tumor are released freely into the circulation, avoiding hepatic clearance.

3. **Carcinoid heart disease** occurs in two-thirds of patients who have the carcinoid syndrome. Tricuspid regurgitation and tricuspid stenosis are the most common manifestations, but also pulmonary stenosis may occur. Left-sided heart disease occurs infrequently—in less than 10% of patients. The preponderance of lesions on the right side of the heart suggests that the heart disease is related to factors secreted into the hepatic vein by liver metastases. This concept is supported by the fact that the anorectic drugs fenfluramine and dexfenfluramine appear to interfere with normal serotonin metabolism and have been associated with similar cardiac valvular lesions. A second manifestation of the carcinoid syndrome is **hypotension**.

4. **Intestinal manifestations** include gastrointestinal bleeding, obstruction, or, with the carcinoid syndrome, patients may develop diarrhea. The most common type of diarrhea is mixed secretory and hypermotility-induced, producing watery stools unresponsive to fasting.

5. **Airway obstruction** from a carcinoid tumor with localized wheezing is one of the more common presentations of this tumor. These airway tumors are very vascular and may present with hemoptysis in addition to localized wheezing.

6. **Asthma**, with significant wheezing, is another manifestation of high levels of serotonin release. In addition to the above-mentioned localized wheezing from an airway lesion, diffuse wheezing may occur due to bronchial hyperreactivity stimulated by the biogenic amines produced by the carcinoid tumor.

7. **Skin manifestations** are part of the classic manifestations of the carcinoid tumor. Patients have intense cutaneous flushing lasting up to several hours. This involves most prominently the face and upper portions of the body. A rare skin manifestation of a carcinoid tumor involving the pancreas or gallbladder is necrolytic erythema. Effective treatment of carcinoid tumors depends on their location and symptoms. Localized disease and airway may respond to surgical resection. Metastatic disease, however, primarily involves treatment of severe symptoms associated with the carcinoid syndrome. Octreotide is a potent inhibitor of hormone secretion by carcinoid cells, and this agent can provide effective control of diarrhea, flushing, and wheezing in as many as 75% of cases.

HYPERCALCEMIA

HyperCALCEMIAS

Hyperparathyroidism

Cancer
Acute renal failure
Lithium
Congenital (familial hypocalciuric hypercalcemia)
Endocrine diseases (Addison's, pheochromocytoma,
  thyrotoxicosis)
Milk alkalai syndrome
Immobilization (exacerbates another underlying
  disorder)
A and D hypervitaminosis
Sarcoid and other granulomatous diseases

Also: thiazide diuretics

Notes

1. Signs and symptoms of hypercalcemia include neuromuscular weakness, abdominal pain, psychiatric disturbance, renal stones, and fractures ("bones, groans, stones, and psychic moans").
2. When hypercalcemia is confirmed (usually by ionized calcium measurement), then a definite diagnosis must be established.
3. Primary hyperparathyroidism is the most common cause of asymptomatic hypercalcemia in an adult. Therapy for this entity depends upon the age of the patient and the presence of complications. Patients under 50 years old routinely undergo surgery. Other indications include:
   a. Elevation of serum calcium more than 0.25–0.40 mmol/L over the upper limit of normal
   b. History of a life-threatening episode such as dehydration
   c. Decreasing renal function
   d. Renal stones
   e. Elevation of urinary calcium > 400 mg/24 hours
   f. Significant reduction of bone mass by noninvasive measurements.
4. Malignancy-associated hypercalcemia may be due to several mechanisms:
   a. Bony invasion (e.g., prostate, breast)

b. Secretion of PTH-related protein (i.e., squamous cell and uroepithelial cancers)

c. Production of osteoclast activating factor, which is probably interleukin-1 (i.e., myeloma)

5. Thiazide diuretics increase calcium reuptake, whereas loop diuretics (furosemide), after proper rehydration, promote calcium excretion.

6. Immobilization does not cause hypercalcemia alone, but may make an occult cause manifest, such as Paget's disease, hyperparathyroidism, or malignancy.

HYPERPHOSPHATEMIA

HIGH PO₄ PARAS

Hypoparathyroidism
Intestinal absorption (vitamin D)
Graves' disease
Hemolysis

Parenteral PO₄
Oncologic/organ infarction

Paraprotein
Addison's
Renal failure
Acidosis
Sarcoidosis/granulomatous disease

N otes

1. Hyperphosphatemia has many causes, which are outlined by the mnemonic "HIGH PO₄ PARAS." Characterized by a high level of phosphorus (HIGH PO₄), one of the primary causes is hypoparathyroidism.

2. Since parathyroid hormone is phosphaturic, hyperphosphatemia is a cardinal feature of **hypoparathyroidism**. A second important mediator in phosphorus homeostasis is vitamin D. Vitamin D enhances **intestinal absorption** of phosphorus, and hyperphosphatemia may be seen with over-medication of vitamin D or in granulomatous diseases, in which there is enhanced conversion of vitamin D to its

active form. Since steroids enhance the excretion of phosphorus into the urine, particularly mineralocorticoids, Addison's disease with its deficiency of steroids can result in hyperphosphatemia. **Graves' disease** and other causes of hyperthyroidism also act to decrease renal excretion of phosphorus. Enhanced cellular release of phosphorus may occur with **tumor lysis syndrome, organ infarction**, or **hemolysis**. Hyperthyroidism also may act to increase cellular release of phosphorus. An acute metabolic or respiratory acidosis causes a cellular shift of phosphorus out of cells, leading to hyperphosphatemia. **Parenteral administration** of intravenous phosphate salts or phospholipid infusions can increase serum phosphorus levels. Abnormal, positively charged serum proteins, which may occur with multiple myeloma, may cause a marked elevation of phosphorus. These proteins seem to have a very high-binding affinity for phosphorus. Finally, **renal failure** is perhaps the most common and important cause of hyperphosphatemia. This is commonly managed with intestinal phosphate-binding resins and dietary restrictions. Phosphorus can be removed by dialysis only to a limited extent.

HYPERPROLACTINEMIA

PROLACTINS

Pregnancy
Renal failure
Oral contraceptives and other medications
Liver failure
Adenoma (prolactin-secreting tumor)
Chest wall disease (including herpes zoster, surgery)
Thyroidal disease (hypothyroidism)
Infiltrative disease of the pituitary (sarcoidosis, histiocytosis X)
Nursing/nipple stimulation
Stalk effect

Notes

1. Normally, prolactin secretion by the pituitary is restrained by hypothalamic dopamine secretion. Thus, any process that disrupts hypothalamic secretion of dopamine or blocks its activity can cause hyperprolactinemia.

2. Hyperprolactinemia causes hypogonadism in men and, rarely, gynecomastia and galactorrhea. It commonly causes hypogonadism, amenorrhea, and galactorrhea in women; hirsutism is rare.

3. Obtain a careful drug history. Drugs that block dopamine synthesis, release, and action include phenothiazines, butyrophenones, metoclopramide, methyldopa, and reserpine. Estrogen stimulation overcomes normal dopaminergic inhibition. This effect is only seen in high-dose estrogen preparations. Estrogen also blocks prolactin action at the breast, preventing lactation.

4. In addition to serum prolactin levels, laboratory evaluation includes thyroid function tests and, in the appropriate setting, renal and liver function tests. Most patients require cranial imaging (MRI).

5. Any process that affects the pituitary stalk ("stalk effect") blocks dopamine secretion, releasing the pituitary from dopaminergic inhibition and resulting in hyperprolactinemia.

HYPERTHYROIDISM

THE TSH

TSH excess
Hamburger thyrotoxicosis (occult hormone intake)
Ectopic thyroid tissue

Thyroid gland hyperfunction
Stimulator of the thyroid gland
Hashimoto's (release of preformed hormone)

Notes

1. "THE TSH" refers to the first test to order when evaluating thyroid function. There are six major mechanisms of hyperthyroidism: (1) TSH excess, (2) "hamburger" thyrotoxicosis/occult source of hormone, (3) ectopic functioning thyroid tissue, (4) thyroid gland hyperfunction, (5) unregulated stimulators of the thyroid gland, and (6) Hashimoto's/release of preformed hormone. Of these mechanisms, the latter three, "TSH," are the most common. TSH is elevated in the first case and suppressed in the other five. In addition to TSH, assays for T3 and T4 function, auto-antibody titers, and possibly scintillation scanning are often indicated.

In acutely ill, hospitalized patients, TSH levels may not reflect thyroid function accurately and cannot be relied on.

2. **TSH excess** is quite rare and is caused by TSH-secreting tumors and scenarios in which the pituitary is resistant to feedback inhibition. **Hamburger thyrotoxicosis** (ingestion of animal thyroid tissue) and surreptitious use of thyroid hormone (thyrotoxicosis factitia) are secondary to an exogenous source of thyroid hormone. **Ectopic thyroid tissue** is a rare condition in which ovarian tissue (struma ovarii) or a metastatic follicular thyroid carcinoma produces excess thyroid hormone. **Thyroid gland hyperfunction** occurs with a hyperfunctioning adenoma and in toxic multinodular goiter. **Stimulators of the thyroid gland** act like TSH, and the most common is the long-acting thyroid stimulator (LATS) of Grave's disease. Trophoblastic tumors may also produce an abnormal thyroid stimulator. **Hashimoto's thyroiditis** as well as irradiation, subacute, and chronic thyroiditis cause hyperthyroidism by excessive leakage of preformed thyroid hormone into the circulation. Thyroid suppressive therapy is useless in these patients, and treatment is aimed at ameliorating the symptoms of thyrotoxicosis.

3. Manifestations of hyperthyroidism include nervousness, emotional lability, inability to sleep, tremors, frequent bowel movements, sweating, weight loss, and heat intolerance. Proximal muscle weakness, tremor, hyperreflexia, tachycardia, hypertension with widened pulse pressure, and other signs of sympathetic overstimulation are characteristic. Grave's disease patients may also demonstrate distinctive infiltrative ophthalmopathy and dermopathy. In a few (usually older) patients, a clinical picture of apathy, weight loss, and hypermetabolism possibly complicated by heart failure and atrial arrhythmias ("apathetic thyrotoxicosis") may be present. A rare syndrome of hypokalemic periodic paralysis may occur in thyrotoxic patients, especially Asian and Latin American men.

4. The following mnemonic lists most of the causes of hyperthyroidism:

I GET A TSH

Irradiation

Graves' disease
Exogenous hyperthyroidism (iodine, iatrogenic, factitious)
Toxic multinodular goiter

Adenoma

TSH-producing tumor
Subacute thyroiditis
Hashimoto's

Also: "TSH" (Trophoblastic disease, Struma ovarii, Heparin—all very rare)

HYPOCALCEMIA

IS PTH OK?

Iatrogenic
Sepsis

Parathyroidectomy/**P**seudohypoparathyroidism
Tumor lysis/**T**rauma
Hypoparathyroidism/**H**ypomagnesemia

Osteomalacia (rickets)
Kidney disease

Notes

1. Hypocalcemia may be a transient phenomena or a chronic condition. Critical to determining the cause of a low measured serum calcium is understanding the functional state of parathyroid hormone (PTH; "IS PTH OK?"). PTH acts to increase serum calcium, and in hypocalcemic states may be present, but transiently dysregulated; absent; present and ineffective; or overwhelmed.

2. When interpreting the serum calcium, remember that a low serum albumin results in a low measurement of serum calcium. An ionized calcium measurement will be normal.

3. **Iatrogenic causes** include transfusions of citrated blood products, plasma exchange therapy, and medications such as heparin, protamine, and glucagon. These effects are usually transient and may not require treatment.

4. **Sepsis** and critical illness often are accompanied by a low serum calcium, but often have normal ionized calcium levels. Pancreatitis causes a persistent low calcium level during the acute stage for unclear reasons. Treatment is probably not indicated in most patients, since the signs and symptoms of hypocalcemia are absent. Remember that IV calcium and hypercalcemic states may precipitate pancreatitis.

5. **Parathyroidectomy**, either intentionally or as a result of thyroid surgery, results in the absence of PTH. The immediate postoperative period presents particular problems if severe bone disease is present. Osteitis fibrosis results from long-standing hyperparathyroidism, and bone mineral deficits are large, resulting in the inability to respond to low serum calcium levels.

6. **Pseudohypoparathyroidism** is a hereditary disease characterized by end-organ unresponsiveness to PTH. PTH is present (in increased amounts) and ineffective. Parathyroid gland hypertrophy is present.

7. **Tumor lysis syndrome** and **trauma causing rhabdomyolysis** are acute causes of hyperphosphatemia, and calcium levels fall precipitously. Concomitant renal failure exacerbates the hyperphosphatemia, and PTH is overwhelmed. Treatment is directed toward lowering phosphorous and improving renal function.

8. **Hypoparathyroidism** can occur as an isolated congenital defect or in association with other anomalies. Acquired hypoparathyroidism may occur after surgery (discussed above) or as an autoimmune phenomenon. PTH is absent or in insufficient amounts.

9. **Hypomagnesemia**, when severe, is associated with hypocalcemia due to impaired PTH release. PTH is absent or inappropriately low.

10. **Osteomalacia** (rickets) occurs when vitamin D is absent (dietary, lack of sunlight, intestinal malabsorption), defectively metabolized (anticonvulsant therapy, vitamin D–dependent rickets type I) or ineffective (liver disease, renal disease, vitamin D–dependent rickets type II). Without vitamin D, PTH is ineffective.

11. **Kidney disease** results in phosphate retention, which lowers calcium and interferes with conversion of 25-OH vitamin D to its active 1,25 OH form. In a sense, it overwhelms PTH and makes it ineffective. Reducing dietary phosphate and using phosphate binders and calcitriol therapy are the cornerstones of treatment.

HYPOGLYCEMIA

INSULINOMAS

Insulinoma
Neoplasm (e.g., large retroperitoneal tumors)
Sulfonylureas
Uremia/renal failure
Liver failure
Insulin antibody syndrome
Nutrition ("reactive hypoglycemia")
Other drugs (ethanol, propranolol, aspirin)
Münchausen's syndrome (self-administered insulin)
Adrenal insufficiency (including panhypopituitarism)
Starvation

Also: rare hereditary enzymatic defects

Notes

1. **Insulin** and **sulfonylurea therapy** cause the great majority of hypoglycemic episodes. A careful assessment of medications is essential, as mistakes in medications may cause hypoglycemia (e.g., acetylhexamide substitution for acetazolamide). **Other medications** can cause symptomatic hypoglycemia such as intravenous pentamadine in AIDS patients. Some drugs may have activity similar to sulfonylureal agents (e.g., Bactrim), causing hypoglycemia in elderly or malnourished patients.

2. Symptoms of hypoglycemia are related to **epinephrine secretion** and **CNS glucose deprivation**. A rapid drop in glucose level leads to symptoms associated with excess epinephrine secretion such as tachycardia, sweating, tremor, anxiety, and hunger. With more gradual drops, CNS symptoms predominate, such as dizziness, headache, clouding of vision, confusion, and seizures.

3. Insulinoma is a rare tumor. Levels of insulin, proinsulin and C-peptide should be obtained during hypoglycemia. Demonstration of low-glucose and high-insulin levels during the hypoglycemic episode is not sufficient evidence for the diagnosis of insulinoma. Factitious hypoglycemia from insulin injection or sulfonylurea drugs is probably the most common cause of hypoglycemia in nondiabetics. Insulin injection causes a rise in insulin levels, but low C-peptide and proinsulin levels. Most patients with insulinomas have elevated proinsulin fractions (> 25% of the total serum insulin). Chronic insulin injection also may induce the development of anti-insulin antibodies.

4. **Pseudohypoglycemia** is a term given to patients who have symptoms 2 to 5 hours after meals, but don't have an associated low glucose level. These patients may be referred for evaluation because of a spuriously low measurement. It should be remembered that approximately 25% of normal individuals have a low serum glucose level 2 to 5 hours after a meal, so this alone is insufficient to diagnose true hypoglycemia. True hypoglycemia should cause symptoms and elicit a hypothalamic-pituitary response of increasing serum cortisol.

5. In the **insulin antibody syndrome**, insulin is bound by the antibodies after a meal. Several hours later, the insulin is released and a hypoglycemic episode occurs.

6. Reactive hypoglycemia may be difficult to diagnose, and oral glucose tolerance testing is not helpful. A high percentage of normal people demonstrate a decrease in serum glucose, since insulin levels normally rise after a meal.

7. Tumors are a rare cause of hypoglycemia, and insulinoma is the most common. Non-islet cell tumors cause hypoglycemia by several mechanisms: (1) release of insulin-like growth factor II (IGF-II) or its high molecular weight precursor ("big" IGF), (2) massive tumor burden with high glucose utilization, (3) hepatic infiltration by tumor, and (4) production of autoantibodies to insulin or its receptor.

HYPOPHOSPHATEMIA

PHOSPHORS

Parathyroidectomy
Hyperventilation
Oncogenic
Starvation-refeeding
Phosphate binders
Hyperthermia
Osteomalacia
Recovery from diabetic ketoacidosis
Steroids

PHOS FATE

Parathyroidectomy
Hyperparathyroidism
Oncogenic
Steroids

Feeding
Alkalosis
Thermal injury/hyperthermia
Enteric (PO_4 binders, dietary deficiency)

1. Hypophosphatemia can be moderate or severe. Severe hypophosphatemia is defined as phosphorus levels in the serum below 0.3 mM/L. The effects of phosphorus depletion include rhabdomyolysis, cardiomyopathy, respiratory failure, erythrocyte dysfunction, leukocyte dysfunction, skeletal demineralization and bone disease, nervous system dysfunction, and metabolic acidosis.
2. Hyperparathyroidism is associated with phosphorus depletion; however, after **parathyroidectomy** for long-standing hyperparathyroidism, "hungry bone syndrome" may occur, and large amounts of phosphorus may go rapidly into the bone, producing clinical hypophosphatemia. **Hyperventilation** results in a respiratory alkalosis. The elevation in pH increases the rate of glycolysis and subsequent phosphorylation of glucose. This results in an immediate cellular uptake of phosphorus and hypophosphatemia. So-called **oncogenic** osteomalacia is a

renal phosphate wasting syndrome associated with certain mesenchymal tumors. It is thought that an as yet unidentified mediator promotes excessive urinary phosphorus loss. **Starvation** with subsequent re-feeding also may result in significant hypophosphatemia in the initial days of calorie repletion. The same effect can be seen with hyperalimentation.

In chronic **alcoholics**, phosphorus content is reduced in skeletal muscles, probably because of renal phosphate losses. When chronic alcoholics go into withdrawal from alcohol, phosphorus may be rapidly taken up into the skeleton, muscle, or liver, resulting in severe hypophosphatemia, which may in turn precipitate acute rhabdomyolysis. Phosphate-binding antacids may decrease intestinal absorption of phosphorus and lead to hypophosphatemia if overused.

In cases of **hyperthermia**, particularly the neuroleptic malignant syndrome, phosphate levels may fall acutely. A similar phenomenon can be seen in the recovery from exhausted exercise or with severe thermal burns. **Osteomalacia** or renal rickets results in renal tubular losses of phosphorus. This results from a deficiency of vitamin D, which normally promotes phosphorus absorption. In patients with **diabetic ketoacidosis**, metabolic acidosis and insulin-deficiency mobilize intracellular phosphate stores and lead to their excretion in the urine. These patients also may have had poor nutritional intake, leading to a lower level of phosphate stores. When insulin is then administered and there is increased glucose entry in the cells, phosphorus also enters the cells, and serum hypophosphatemia may result. Finally, **steroid therapy**, particularly aldosterone, but also glucocorticoids, tends to promote phosphate excretion into the urine and may lead to a depletion of total body phosphorus.

3. Treatment of hypophosphatemia depends on the clinical scenario. In acute symptomatic hypophosphatemia, phosphorus salts may be given by intravenous injection. In cases with coexistent hypokalemia, potassium salt may be administered. In treating alcoholics—who often are phosphate-, potassium-, and magnesium-deficient—potassium salt and magnesium sulfate may be coadministered along with glucose.

Syndrome of Inappropriate Antidiuretic Hormone Secretion

SIADH

Small cell carcinoma and other cancers (pancreatic, Hodgkin's disease, thyroid, duodenal)
Infections (tuberculosis, pneumonia, lung abscess)
ARDS/mechanical ventilation/pulmonary disease
Drugs
Head trauma/neurologic disease

Notes

1. SIADH is the term applied to excessive vasopressin release associated with hyponatremia without edema. Urine is inappropriately concentrated (usually > 300 mmol/L) despite a low plasma osmolality and serum sodium concentration. Sodium excretion in the urine is maintained (usually > 20 mmol/L) by hypervolemia, suppression of the renin-angiotensin-aldosterone system, and increased levels of atrial naturietic peptide. BUN and creatinine may decrease due to dilution.

2. SIADH may be secondary to malignancies, pulmonary diseases, drugs, and central nervous system disorders. **Malignancies** causing SIADH include small cell carcinoma, pancreatic carcinoma, Hodgkin's disease, thyroid carcinoma, and duodenal carcinoma. **Pulmonary diseases** causing SIADH include tuberculosis, pneumonia, and lung abscess, as well as chronic obstructive pulmonary disease, ARDS, and mechanical ventilation. **Drugs** that may cause SIADH include hypoglycemic agents, psychotropics, narcotics, and chemotherapeutic agents. **Central nervous system disorders** causing SIADH include head trauma, hemorrhage, encephalitis, meningitis, Guillain-Barré, and porphyria. Other causes of euvolemic hyponatremia include psychogenic polydipsia, hypothyroidism, adrenal insufficiency, pain, surgery, and anesthesia.

3. SIADH should be suspected when patients have hyponatremia and a concentrated urine (> 300 mmol/kg) in the absence of dehydration. Important

conditions to rule out include dilutional hyponatremia (such as occurs in adreno-corticosteroid insufficiency), edematous states (CHF, hypothyroidism), hypertensive states (renal artery stenosis), diuretic use, "pseudohyponatremia" (excessive plasma triglycerides or proteins), and primary polydipsia (always associated with a dilute urine, osmolality < 150 mmol/kg).

4. A water load test as well as urinary or plasma AVP levels are useful in the evaluation. In the water load test, a patient drinks a large volume of fluid and then urine is collected in hourly samples. Normally, at least 65% of the water should be excreted by 4 hours, or 80% by 5 hours, and the lowest urine osmolality (usually reached in the second hour) should be less than 100 mmol/kg. Plasma AVP is immeasurable in hyponatremic states, but in SIADH it is detectable even after a water load.

5. Treatment of SIADH involves relieving the underlying cause and fluid restriction. The drug demeclocycline inhibits ADH and may be a useful treatment. Some patients with chronic SIADH can be treated with a high salt and protein diet. The high osmolarity will increase free water excretion.

VII

NEPHROLOGY

General Considerations

There are two ways of approaching renal disease: (1) based on etiology, as outlined in the MEDICINE DOC mnemonic, and (2) based on pathology from a renal biopsy. It is important to recognize that the same disease process can cause different pathological processes in the kidney (for example, systemic lupus erythematosus may cause a variety of renal lesions).

Metabolic—e.g., amyloidosis, hyperuricemia

Endocrine—e.g., hypercalcemia, hyper and hypothyroidism, SIADH and diabetes insipidus

Drugs/medicines—e.g., chemotherapeutic agents, antibiotics, radiocontrast dye

Infection—e.g., HIV-related, tuberculosis, pyelonephritis

Congenital—polycystic kidney disease, Alport's syndrome, reflux nephropathy

Immunologic—e.g., Goodpasture's, Wegener's granulomatosis, SLE

Neoplastic—e.g., renal cell carcinoma, transitional cell carcinoma, tumor lysis syndrome

Exotic diseases—e.g., sarcoidosis, ITP, cryoglobulinemia

Degenerative—aging, ?hypertension

Occupational/environmental—trauma

Cardiovascular—e.g., atherosclerosis, hypertensive nephropathy, cholesterol emboli

A multitude of **metabolic disorders** may cause renal disease. These include amyloidosis, hypercalcemia, and other diseases that lead to abnormal increases in metabolic products in the blood stream. Hyperlipidemia leading to atherosclerosis also could be considered a metabolic disease leading to renal insufficiency.

Endocrine diseases may be made manifest by renal insufficiency. Again, hypercalcemia, secondary to hyperparathyroidism, can lead to renal failure and/or nephrolithiasis. Diabetes can cause proteinuria or progressive renal insufficiency and, ultimately, renal failure. Other endocrine syndromes involving the kidney include SIADH and hypo- and hyperthyroidism. In addition, renal cell carcinoma may have several associated paraneoplastic syndromes.

Drugs are a frequent cause of renal insufficiency, and virtually any drug can cause renal disease. A common problem is renal insufficiency induced by antihypertensive agents, especially ACE-inhibitors. Other forms of drug-induced renal disease include interstitial nephritis and forms secondary to chemotherapeutic agents, intravenous radiocontrast, or intravenous drug abuse.

Many types of **infections** cause renal disease. HIV disease can lead to severe proteinuria and renal failure. Tuberculosis may primarily involve the kidneys and the urinary tract. Pyelonephritis is also a common infectious disease involving the kidneys.

Congenital diseases can cause renal manifestations. Anomalies of the urinary tract and chronic reflux nephropathy may lead to renal failure. Polycystic kidney disease and medullary sponge kidney disease are familial causes of renal failure. Other inherited metabolic diseases such as Fabry's disease and various storage diseases can lead to renal insufficiency. A variety of congenital disorders may cause renal stones, including cystinosis and Lesch-Nyhan syndrome.

Immunologic diseases often affect the kidneys, and renal disease may be the first manifestation of an immunologic disease. Virtually all of the collagen-vascular diseases (e.g., SLE) have renal manifestations. The vasculitides, including Wegener's, Goodpasture's, and polyarteritis nodosa, may lead to renal failure.

Neoplastic disease may arise primarily in the kidneys or involve the kidneys secondarily. Renal cell carcinoma can be widely metastatic and often has associated paraneoplastic syndromes. Metastatic tumors or locally invasive tumors, often gynecologic, may cause compression of the ureters and renal failure. Hypercalcemia secondary to malignant disease can lead to renal failure, as can multiple myeloma.

Numerous **exotic** diseases affect the kidneys, including sarcoidosis, familial Mediterranean fever, and ITP. Some of these diseases are thought to have an immunologic basis.

Perhaps the most important aspect of **degenerative** disease to consider is the effect of aging on renal function. The glomerular filtration rate decreases steadily with age, and a low serum creatinine may not reflect actual renal function in an elderly patient.

Occupational and environmental exposures may lead to renal dysfunction. Extrinsic trauma can cause kidney damage, hematuria, or frank bleeding. Hydrocarbon exposure may cause Goodpasture's syndrome.

Cardiovascular diseases may involve the kidneys secondarily. Chronic hypertension can lead to renal insufficiency and, ultimately, renal failure. Cholesterol emboli may occur with severe atherosclerotic disease after a radiographic dye procedure. Also, congestive heart failure is a very common cause of pre-renal azotemia.

Edema

THE LEAK OF VEINS or VALVES

Venous disease (obstruction, insufficiency)
Albuminuria/albumin loss in stool
Lymphatic obstruction (congenital, acquired)
Volume overload
Electrolyte/nutritional deficiency
Sepsis/capillary leak

or

Tumor
Heart failure
Enteropathy (protein-losing)

Liver failure
Endocrine (hypothyroidism, aldosteronism, diabetes)
Altitude sickness
Kidney disease (renal failure, nephrotic syndrome)

Obstruction of lymphatics
Filariasis

Venous thrombosis
Eclampsia/pregnancy
Iatrogenic
Nutritional deficiency
Sepsis/capillary leak

Note

"VALVES" refers to the loss of venous valvular competence with aging, a common cause of edema. Edema may result from venous disease (thrombosis, extrinsic compression, trauma, venous valvular insufficiency), loss of albumin (nephrosis, protein-losing enteropathy), lymphatic obstruction (congenital, malignant, filariasis), volume overload (CHF, renal failure, cirrhosis), electrolyte/nutritional deficiencies that cause a loss of venous integrity, and sepsis and other systemic conditions causing capillary leak.

HEMATURIA

UA RBCS

Urethra
Artifactual (e.g., dark urine, menses, medications)

Renal (e.g., trauma, cysts, pyelonephritis)
Bladder
Collecting system
Systemic disorder (e.g., vasculitis, coagulopathy)

Notes

1. Hematuria is defined as the presence of gross blood or RBCs (> 1–2 per hpf) in the spun urinary sediment. It is important initially to look at the sediment to rule out false hematuria. Certain medications (rifampin, phenazopyridine) and diseases (porphyria) may alter urine color. Also, both myoglobinuria and hemoglobinuria cause a positive dipstick test with a negative urinary sediment. Menstruation also can be mistaken for hematuria.
2. Hematuria may originate at any site from glomerulus to the urethra. The presence of "crenated" RBCs, RBC casts, proteinuria, or elevated BUN and creatinine support a glomerular source. Isolated hematuria (without casts or proteinuria) suggests bleeding from a site in the collecting system, bladder, or urethra. Possibilities include neoplasms, TB, renal stones, trauma, papillary necrosis, analgesic neopathy, prostatitis, cystitis, or urethritis.
3. Initially, exclude UTI, coagulation disorders, and TB. The patient's age and presentation determine the direction of the work-up. For example, a young female with dysuria would most likely be treated with a trial of antibiotics, while an older man with recent onset of gross hematuria may be investigated with renal imaging and/or cystoscopy. In younger patients without evidence of infection, an IVP is often the first imaging test ordered.

4. A common renal disease that features hematuria is IgA nephropathy. IgA nephropathy is characterized by gross or microscopic hematuria without other symptoms. The prognosis is variable, but disease progression typically is slow, with approximately 50% of patients developing renal failure within 23 years of diagnosis. Self-limited acute renal failure may develop following an upper respiratory infection. There is no known effective treatment for IgA nephropathy, and the role of renal biopsy in this disorder is controversial.

5. Some of the more common causes of hematuria are summarized by the following mnemonic:

I PEE RBCS

Infection

Pseudohematuria (menses, dark urine)
Exercise
External trauma

Renal disease (glomerular source)
Benign prostatic hypertrophy
Cancer
Stones

6. Here is a more complete differential for hematuria:

I'D PASS HEMATURIA

IgA nephropathy
Drugs/dark urine (pseudohematuria)

Polycystic kidney disease
Analgesic nephropathy
Sickle cell
Stones

Hemoglobinuria, myoglobinuria, porphyria
Exercise
Malignancy
Acute glomerulonephritis
Trauma
Urethritis
Renal infarction
Infection
Alport's syndrome and other inherited diseases
    (e.g., sickle cell, polycystic kidney disease)

HYPERTENSION

I CHECK A BP

Idiopathic (essential)

CNS disorders
High output states
Endocrine diseases
Coarctation
Kidney disease

Acute stress

Birth control pills and other drugs
Pregnancy

Note

Essential hypertension accounts for greater than 90% of hypertension cases. The primary causes of an elevated blood pressure are outlined by "I CHECK A BP."

Secondary Hypertension

RENALS

Renal
Endocrine
Neurologic
Aortic coarctation
Licorice gluttony
Scleroderma

Notes

1. Hypertension is idiopathic, "essential," or secondary to one of the causes outlined by "RENALS."
2. **Renal diseases** that cause hypertension include many types of renal parenchymal disease as well as renovascular hypertension.
3. **Endocrine causes** of secondary hypertension are acromegaly, aldosteronism, J-G cell tumor, Cushing's syndrome, pheochromocytoma, and hypercalcemia. Pheochromocytomas are characterized by paroxysmal or sustained episodes of severe hypertension. Headache, palpitations, and/or profuse diaphoresis are almost always associated with the hypertension. The tumors may secrete epinephrine, norepinephrine, serotonin, or nothing. The "ten percent rule" refers to the observation that 10% are malignant, 10% are bilateral, and 10% are extra-adrenal. Extra-adrenal sites include sympathetic ganglia (organ of Zuckerkandel) and the bladder (micturition-associated symptoms). A J-G cell tumor produces renin leading to hypertension. It may resemble Conn's syndrome (primary hyperaldosteronism), except that renin levels are decreased in Conn's syndrome. Oral contraceptives could be considered an exogenous endocrine cause of secondary hypertension. Estrogens stimulate angiotensinogen production by the liver, thereby increasing angiotensin II and aldosterone levels. Steroid therapy also raises blood pressure.
4. **Neurologic disorders** causing hypertension include increased intracranial pressure, acute spinal cord injury, dysautonomia, polyneuritis (acute porphyria, lead poisoning), and psychogenic factors.
5. **Aortic coarctation** may be diagnosed by a blood pressure and pulse differential between upper and lower extremities and characteristic rib-notching (from increased flow through intercostal arteries) seen on x-ray.
6. **Licorice** contains glycyrrhizic acid, which increases the mineralocorticoid effects of endogenous cortisol.
7. **Scleroderma** renal crisis is a dramatic and life-threatening manifestation of the disease. ACE inhibitors are the treatment of choice.

HYPERKALEMIA

A HI K

Acidosis

Hypoaldosteronism
Iatrogenic/Inaccurate measurement (LAB error, drugs, IV potassium)

Kidney disease (renal failure, renal tubular disease)

Notes

1. The primary causes of a high serum potassium are summarized by "A HI K." **Acidosis** causes potassium to shift out of cells. **Hypoaldosteronism** causes hyperkalemia because aldosterone normally promotes renal potassium excretion. **Iatrogenic** causes of hyperkalemia include drug therapy (heparin, potassium-sparing diuretics) and IV solutions containing potassium. **Inaccurate measurements** may be obtained when hemolysis of the specimen occurs or from poor blood drawing technique (overinflation of blood pressure cuff). Finally, **kidney disease** inhibits normal potassium excretion and leads to hyperkalemia.

2. True hyperkalemia occurs by one of three mechanisms: **inadequate excretion** (renal disease, hypovolemia, hypoaldosteronism, potassium-sparing diuretics), **potassium shift** from tissues (tissue damage, drugs, acidosis, hyperosmolality, insulin deficiency, hyperkalemic periodic paralysis), or **excessive intake**. Pseudo-hyperkalemia occurs with thrombocytosis, leukocytosis, or in vitro hemolysis.

3. Renal mechanisms of hyperkalemia involve a decrease in filtered blood or tubular disease. Acute renal failure is more likely to cause severe hyperkalemia than chronic renal insufficiency, unless oliguria supervenes. Hyporeninemic hypoaldosteronism may be seen in patients with moderate renal dysfunction. Type IV renal tubular acidosis, frequently seen in diabetics as well as other interstitial nephritides, is associated with a hyperchloremic metabolic acidosis. Nonsteroidal anti-inflammatory drugs, converting enzyme inhibitors, and beta-blockers may induce hypoperinemic hypoaldosteronism.

4. Drugs that may induce hyperkalemia include heparin (inhibits aldosterone secretion), potassium-sparing diuretics, succinylcholine, digitalis, and arginine, as well as NSAIDs, ACE inhibitors, and beta-blockers.

5. Artifactual elevation of potassium may occur if blood is drawn after repeated clenching of the fist and tourniquet application. For this reason, always immediately recheck an elevated potassium level.

6. Management should involve an immediate EKG to look for high-peaked T waves, prolongation of the PR interval, or complete heart block. Progressive hyperkalemia leads to a "sinewave" EKG configuration, ventricular fibrillation, and standstill. Acute interventions include administration of IV calcium (which is cardioprotective) as well as IV insulin, glucose, bicarbonate, and possibly epinephrine, all of which shift potassium intracellularly. Potassium-binding resins, diuretics, and/or dialysis may be indicated to remove potassium from the body.

7. Here is a more complete list of the causes of hyperkalemia:

A BAD K PLIGHT

Aldosterone deficiency (Addison's congenital adrenal hyperplasia, hyporeninemia, heparin)

Blood diseases (thrombocytosis, leukocytosis, leukemia)
Acidosis
Drugs

Kidney disease (renal failure, renal tubular disease)

Periodic paralysis (hyperkalemic)
Laboratory error
Intravenous potassium administration, antibiotics
Geophagia/excessive intake
Hyperosmolality
Tissue necrosis

Hypernatremia

AVP

Altered mental status/abnormal thirst/access to water
  impaired
Volume loss (renal, extra-renal)
Primary sodium gain (rare, iatrogenic)

Notes

Arginine vasopressin (AVP) is also called antidiuretic hormone, and its major action is to conserve water by concentrating the urine. AVP release is primarily regulated by changes in concentration of plasma solutes. As plasma osmolality rises, so do the levels of AVP. To a lesser extent, decreases in plasma volume also stimulate the release of AVP. Water deprivation causes both hyperosmolality and volume depletion, and thus is a potent stimulus to AVP release. AVP then acts to maximally concentrate the urine, thus defending volume. The loss of effective AVP leads to volume loss and hypernatremia.

1. Hypernatremia is defined as a serum sodium of greater than 145 mM/L. Since sodium and its accompanying anions are the major effective osmols of the extracellular fluid, **hypernatremia is by definition a state of hyperosmolality**. The three major mechanisms of hypernatremia are outlined by the AVP mnemonic: (1) altered mental status or impaired access to free water; (2) volume loss; (3) primary sodium gain. In the strictest sense, either free water is lost, which is the most common scenario, or, more rarely, total sodium is gained. The appropriate response to hypovolemia and hypernatremia is increasing water intake (stimulated by thirst) and excreting a maximally concentrated urine (controlled by AVP release).
2. Most cases of hypernatremia are secondary to a net loss of free water. **Altered mental status** in acutely ill or post-operative patients, limited **access** in infants, handicapped patients and mechanically ventilated patients, and **abnormal thirst mechanism** in patients with a hypothalamic injury all cause a net loss of free water. Hypothalamic impairment may be due to granulomatous disease, tumors, cerebrovascular accident, or, rarely, "essential hypernatremia." Essential hypernatremia represents an osmo-receptor defect in AVP release. It is characterized by a lack of response to forced water intake.
3. **Volume depletion** from free water losses may be either renal or extra-renal. Renal free water losses are most commonly secondary to drugs, such as loop

diuretics, which interfere with counter-current reabsorption. An osmotic diuresis also may result in net-free water loss. Hyperglycemia from uncontrolled diabetes is the most common cause; however, Mannitol administration has the same result. Increased urea levels from a high-protein diet or steroid therapy can result in an osmotic diuresis and net-free water loss.

When there is a loss of AVP function, the syndrome of diabetes insipidus results. There are two primary categories of diabetes insipidus: central diabetes insipidus, which results from destruction of the neurohypophysis and thus the neurons which secrete AVP, and nephrogenic diabetes, which entails a lack of responsiveness of the kidney to AVP. This may be either a primary congenital defect or secondary to lithium administration, hypercalcemia, hypokalemia, papillary necrosis, or pregnancy. Pregnancy is an interesting physiological state, in that the placenta secretes a vasopressinase, which decreases the effective activity of AVP.

4. Lastly, **primary sodium gain** may lead to hypernatremia. However, this is rare and iatrogenic. Most commonly, this results from administration of hypertonic saline or sodium bicarbonate solutions in hospitalized patients.

5. Like hyponatremia, patients with hypernatremia can be divided into hypovolemic, euvolemic, and hypervolemic categories. **Hypovolemic hypernatremia** occurs in the very young and very old, and is seen in situations of extreme extracellular fluid losses and/or an inability to take in free water adequately (febrile illnesses, vomiting, diarrhea, and severe renal losses). **Euvolemic hypernatremia** also can be due to extracellular fluid loss without adequate access to water, or from the loss of control of water homeostasis. Diabetes insipidus, either central or nephrogenic, causes an inability to reabsorb filtered water, resulting in systemic hypertonicity but a hyperosmolar urine. **Hypervolemic hypernatremia**, although uncommon, is iatrogenic, and it may occur after sodium bicarbonate injection or administration of hypertonic saline.

6. For the great majority of patients, the treatment of hypernatremia initially involves volume repletion with hypotonic fluids. Normal saline is relatively hypotonic, but should only be used to establish circulatory stability. Once circulatory stability is attained, patients can then be rehydrated either intravenously or (preferably) orally with more hypotonic fluids. Be careful to *slowly* correct the water deficit—no more than 12 mEq/L over 24 hours. Cerebral edema may result from too rapid correction.

7. In choosing the appropriate fluids for correction, it is critical to know the patient's urinary concentrating capacity. Some patients, especially those with diabetes insipidus, have urinary osmolalities as low as 40 to 60 mmol/L. An infusion of half-normal saline (osmolality 154 mmol/L) will result in a further rise in serum sodium, and so more hypotonic fluids (5% dextrose in water) should be administered. In some cases of central diabetes insipidus, a synthetic analog of antidiuretic hormone, DDAVP, can be administered either intravenously or intranasally.

8. Helpful formulas for correcting total body sodium and water deficits are available in the *New England Journal of Medicine*, Vol. 342(20):1497, 2000. To estimate the effect of 1 L of any infusate on the serum osmolality, use the following formula:

$$\text{Change in serum Na}^+ = \frac{[\text{infusate Na}^+ - \text{serum Na}^+]}{[\text{total body water (liters)} + 1]}$$

Total body water is usually estimated as 40–60% of the body weight (0.4–0.6 × wt. in kg). This formula allows you to predict the effect of 1 L of a particular intravenous fluid on the serum sodium. To decide how much fluid to give, simply divide the desired correction (e.g., 12 mEq/24 hrs) by the change in serum Na$^+$ calculated by the equation. Also add to this amount extra volume for ongoing losses during the infusion time. This approach works well for most causes of free water loss as long as the change in electrolyte concentrations and ongoing free water are carefully monitored. As mentioned above, the individual patient's urinary concentrating ability must be known (urine osmolality).

9. AVP conserves water by concentrating the urine. It increases the permeability of the distal collecting duct, thereby facilitating free water reuptake into the medullary interstitium. In the absence of AVP, free water is lost and hypernatremia ensues. The causes of hypernatremia are organized by the following mnemonic. "TIGHT COLLECTOR" refers to an impermeable collecting duct (lack of effective AVP activity) and subsequent free water losses, and "A STUPID MD" refers to the often iatrogenic causes of primary sodium gain.

TIGHT COLLECTOR VS. A STUPID MD

Low AVP 2° to CNS disease
Trauma
Infection (meningitis, encephalitis, etc.)
Guillain-Barré
Hemorrhage
Tumor/mass

Ineffective AVP 2° to renal impairment
Congenital nephrogenic diabetes insipidus
Osmotic diuresis
Lithium/drugs
Loop diuretics
Early phase of ATN (polyuric)
Calcium elevation
Tubular defect (especially medullary cystic kidney)
Other intrinsic renal diseases
Relief of urinary obstruction

Nonrenal free water losses
Vomiting/diarrhea/NG suction
Skin/sweating

Inadequate intake
Altered mental status/altered thirst/access impairment

Primary sodium gain
Saline infusion (hypertonic relative to concentrating ability)
TPN
Uterine injection with hypertonic saline
PO salt
IV bicarbonate
Dialysate (hypertonic)

Mineralocorticoids (Cushing's, Conn's)
Drowning, drinking sea water

Hypokalemia

LESS K

Lasix/diuretics
Enteric losses (e.g., diarrhea, fistulas)
Steroids (Cushing's, aldosteronism, exogenous steroids)
Shift (alkalosis, treatment of DKA, periodic paralysis)

Kidney disease (renal tubular acidosis [RTA], Liddle's syndrome)

A MEGA K DROP

Alkalosis

Magnesium depletion
Enteric losses (diarrhea)
Glucocorticoid excess (Cushing's, exogenous steroids, ectopic ACTH)
Aldosteronism

Ketoacidosis

Diuretics (thiazides, furosemide, ethacrynic acid)
Rental tubular diseases (RTA, Liddle's, leukemia, antibiotics)
Osmotic diuresis
Periodic paralysis

Notes

1. The principle mechanisms of hypokalemia are:
    a. Enteric losses
    b. Kidney losses (RTA, diuretics, osmotic diuresis, mineralocorticoids and glucocorticoid excess, magnesium deficiency)
    c. Shift of cellular potassium (alkalosis, periodic paralysis, insulin effect, catecholamines)

2. **Enteric losses** are usually due to diarrhea, although vomiting, villous adenomas, fistulas, and uretosigmoidostomy may lead to excessive potassium loss. With vomiting, loss of gastric acid leads to metabolic alkalosis, which increases tubular bicarbonate concentration. Increases in bicarbonate anions eventuate in increased tubular potassium concentration and subsequent excretion. In addition, secondary hyperaldosteronism from volume depletion contributes to potassium losses.

3. **Kidney losses** can occur with volume concentration and metabolic alkalosis, diuretic use and osmotic diuresis, excess mineralocorticoid activity, or in renal tubular disease. Diuretics augment sodium and fluid delivery to the distal tubule potassium secretory site, thereby enhancing potassium losses. In osmotic diuresis, such as in diabetic ketoacidosis, excessive potassium losses occur due to urinary losses of negatively charged keto acids. The serum potassium may be normal initially due to cellular shift, but it falls precipitously with correction of the acidosis.

Excessive mineralocorticoid activity can be seen with primary aldosteronism, or with secondary aldosteronism in conjunction with malignant hypertension, Bartter's syndrome, and juxtaglomerular cell tumors. Licorice contains glycerrhizic acid, which inhibits 11-B-hydroxysteroid dehydrogenase. This enzyme converts cortisol to an inactive form with no mineralocorticoid activity. Inhibition of the enzyme increases the mineralocorticoid activity of endogenous cortisol.

Glucocorticoids stimulate renal potassium secretion, leading to hypokalemia and alkalosis. Renal tubular potassium wasting occurs in types I and II renal tubular acidosis, Liddle's syndrome, leukemia-associated renal tubular disease, and in tubular dysfunction secondary to drug therapy (penicillins, amphotericin B).

4. Hypokalemia also is seen in conditions that cause an **intracellular shift** of potassium, such as alkalosis, periodic paralysis, insulin administration, or increased beta-adrenergic activity. This shift is the premise for treating hyperkalemia with insulin, glucose, bicarbonate, and beta-adrenergic agents.

5. Iatrogenic causes such as **lasix-diuretic administration** and **steroid therapy** are common in renal potassium loss.

6. The presence of hypertension suggests hyperaldosteronism or glucocorticoid excess. In Bartter's syndrome, there is secondary hyperaldosteronism, but normal blood pressure. A high renin level supports the diagnosis of a renin-secreting tumor. In normotensive patients, urinary potassium levels should be assessed. Low urinary potassium excretion suggests GI losses or prior diuretic use. High urinary potassium (> 25 mmol/L) suggests renal tubular acidosis, diabetic ketoacidosis, vomiting, current diuretic use, or Bartter's syndrome.

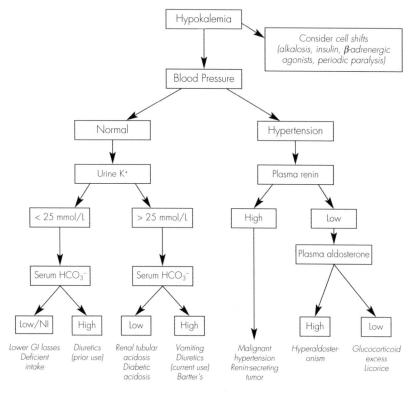

Flow chart for hypokalemia evaluation. (From Levinsky NG: Fluids and electrolytes. In Isselbacher, Braunwald, Wilsen, et al. (eds): Harrison's Principles of Internal Medicine, 13th ed. New York, McGraw-Hill, 1994; with permission.)

HYPONATREMIA

OSM

Osmotically active solute
Sodium disorder
Measurement error

Notes

1. The serum **osmolality** and the patient's **volume status** are the two key elements in evaluating the cause of a low serum sodium. Hyponatremia (sodium < 135 mEq/L) does not simply indicate a state of low total body sodium. Total body sodium may be reduced, normal, or increased. The measured serum sodium concentration is dependent on the serum osmolality ("OSM"), which determines whether a pathologic sodium disorder is present. A serum osmolality differentiates between the three categories of hyponatremia: (1) Osmotically active solutes, (2) Sodium disorders, and (3) Measurement errors.

2. A high serum osmolality (> 285) indicates the presence of osmotically active solutes such as mannitol or glucose. Glucose and mannitol are **osmotically active solutes**, which cause water movement out of cells and a dilution of the plasma. Hyponatremia ensues but, since plasma osmolality is increased, clinical manifestations of hypotonicity are absent. The low serum sodium is, in a sense, appropriate, since a normal sodium level would lead to an even higher osmolality. This scenario is commonly encountered in patients with hyperglycemia, in whom correction of the high glucose levels with insulin is accompanied by a rise in serum sodium. An osmotic diuresis causes free water loss, and hypernatremia may result after clearing the osmotically active solute.

3. A pathologic **sodium disorder** is defined by a low serum osmolality (< 280), the causes of which may be divided into hypovolemic, euvolemic, and hypervolemic etiologies as listed on pages 148–149.

4. A normal serum osmolality (280–285) suggests pseudohyponatremia due to a **measurement error**, which can occur in severe hyperlipidemia or hyperproteinemia. This type of error is less common with newer laboratory techniques.

5. Once pseudohyponatremia from measurement errors and accumulation of osmotically active solutes is ruled out, then a true, pathologic sodium disorder is present. The patient's volume status is then used to elucidate the cause. Edematous states and profound volume depletion are usually obvious, but in some cases it may be difficult to distinguish between moderate volume depletion, normovolemia, and modest volume expansion by physical examination alone.

6. Hypovolemic hyponatremia indicates salt losses in excess of water losses. If a hyponatremic patient appears to be clinically volume depleted, then it should be determined whether the losses are **extra-renal** (sequestration or skin) or **renal** (osmotically active solutes, diuretic therapy, urinary salt wasting, dopamine infusion or mineralocorticoid deficiency). Measurement of the urinary sodium establishes the cause, with a high urine sodium (> 20 mmol/L) indicating renal losses, and a low urine sodium (< 10 mmol/L) indicating renal sodium conservation and extra-renal losses.

7. Euvolemic hyponatremia is essentially a result of **excessive free water intake** (with inadequate solute intake), or **excessive ADH activity**. Excessive, surreptitious, free water intake occurs with psychiatric illnesses. This condition may be difficult to distinguish from SIADH, since patients do not acknowledge the problem. Other forms of this intake imbalance are "beer potomania," an excessive intake of hypotonic fluids with little dietary solute, and the "tea and toast" syndrome, in which elderly patients inadvertently have a similar dietary imbalance. The latter problem may be made manifest when a diuretic is prescribed to an elderly patient with a poor diet. Elevated ADH levels inhibit the kidney from excreting free water. The result is modest volume expansion (often clinically inapparent) and hyponatremia.

The key feature of SIADH is an inappropriately concentrated urine in the face of serum hypo-osmolality and normovolemia. There are many causes of SIADH, including drugs, neoplasms, and CNS disorders. Some other states such as pain, emotion, and the postoperative state may also temporarily impair water excretion, probably as a result of an ADH-mediated mechanism. ADH is probably important in endocrine causes of hyponatremia such as hypothyroidism and pure cortisol deficiency (Addison's disease usually results in hypovolemia and features salt-wasting). In SIADH, urine sodium usually exceeds 20 mmol/L unless fluid intake has been restricted.

8. An important distinction to make in neurosurgical patients is between SIADH and cerebral salt wasting (a hypovolemic state). Cerebral salt wasting is relatively rare and may be related to elevated levels of atrial natriuretic peptide (ANP). The diagnosis depends on establishing a reduction in blood volume and inappropriate natriuresis. Volume restriction (as is appropriate in SIADH) may be hazardous in cerebral salt wasting since it can lead to cerebral ischemia from vasospasm. The proper treatment is to maintain intravascular volume and correct hyponatremia with normal saline infusion. Dopamine also stimulates ANP release and promotes natriuresis.

9. A less well understood euvolemic state is "essential" hyponatremia or the "sick cell" syndrome. It is hypothesized that these patients have a **reset serum "osmostat"** (< 280 mmol/L) and maintain a lower serum sodium due to reestablishing the "normal" range of osmolality. Alternatively, it may also represent a state of elevated ADH activity secondary to an unknown nonosmotic stimulus. When osmolality is lowered sufficiently, osmotic inhibition of ADH overcomes the nonosmotic stimulus.

10. Hypervolemic hyponatremia occurs with edematous states. Mechanistically, these conditions are similar to the hypovolemic states in that the effective circulating volume is reduced and the kidney conserves sodium (urine sodium < 10 mmol/L). CHF is the most common cause of hypervolemic hyponatremia, and hyponatremia is associated with a poor prognosis. Loss of plasma proteins (albuminuria, protein-losing enteropathy) causes third spacing of fluids, intravascular depletion, and hyponatremia. End-stage liver disease impairs circulation and plasma protein synthesis with consequent edema and hyponatremia. Renal failure impairs the ability to excrete a normal volume of dilute urine and results in hyponatremia and edema. Early in the course of renal failure, the volume expansion may be modest, and patients may appear to have euvolemic hyponatremia.

11. Treatment: In general, only severe, symptomatic hyponatremia and hyponatremia developing over 24 hours or less (e.g., patients with psychogenic polydipsia, surgical and obstetric patients) should be treated with hypertonic solution and more prompt correction. In the majority of patients, **rapid correction of hyponatremia is hazardous and may lead to central nervous system damage** (i.e., central pontine myelinolysis). A standard rule is that the serum sodium should not be raised by more than 0.5 to 1.0 mmol/L per hour and **no more than 12 mmol/L over 24 hours**. Another maxim of hyponatremia treatment is that the time for correction should approximate the time course of development (i.e., rapidly occurring hyponatremia should be corrected rapidly, and more chronic conditions should be corrected gradually).

12. The following mnemonic separates hyponatremic conditions into four categories: **pseudohyponatremia**, and **hypovolemic, euvolemic,** and **hypervolemic** (edematous) states:

A SODIUM WATER CAPER

Pseudohyponatremia
Artifactual

Hypovolemic
Sequestration, **S**kin losses (burns and sweating)
Osmotic diuresis
Diuretics
Intestinal losses (diarrhea, vomiting)
Urinary salt wasting
Mineralocorticoid deficiency

Euvolemic
Water intoxication
ADH excess (SIADH)
Temporary impairment of water excretion (pain, emotion, drugs, post-operative)
Endocrine (hypothyroidism, pure cortisol deficiency)
Reset osmostat ("sick cell")

Hypervolemic
Congestive heart failure
Albuminuria
Protein-losing enteropathy
End-stage liver disease (cirrhosis)
Renal failure

NEPHROTIC SYNDROME

MAD NEPHROTICS

Medications/toxins/drugs
Amyloidosis
Diabetes

Neoplasm
Endocarditis/infections
Primary glomerular disease
Hereditary diseases
Renal vein thrombosis
Obesity (morbid)
Thyroid disease (myxedema and thyroiditis)
Interstitial nephritis
Chronic reflux/obstruction
SLE, collagen vascular diseases

Notes

1. Nephrotic syndrome is characterized by albuminuria (> 3.5 g/d), hypo-albuminemia, and edema. Urinary loss of critical plasma proteins predisposes patients to thromboembolic events (renal vein thrombosis, pulmonary embolus), hyperlipidemia and accelerated atherosclerosis, vitamin D deficiency, and protein malnutrition, as well as drug toxicity from decreased plasma protein binding.
2. The majority of cases are due to glomerular disease (75%), including membranous (40%), minimal change disease, focal glomerulosclerosis, membrane proliferative glumerulonephritis (GN), and mesangioproliferative GN.

3. Systemic diseases, including diabetes mellitus, SLE, amyloidosis, drug reactions, thyroid disease, infections, and malignancy, as well as obesity, account for about 25% of cases.

4. Malignancies that may be associated with nephrosis include myeloma, Hodgkin's and non-Hodgkin's lymphomas, leukemia, and breast and GI tract carcinomas.

5. Drugs that cause the nephrotic syndrome include gold, heroin, penicillamine, probenicid, captopril, and NSAIDs.

6. Infections associated with the nephrotic syndrome include endocarditis, hepatitis B, shunt infections, syphilis, and malaria.

7. Evaluation of nephrotic syndrome includes 24-hour urine for protein and creatine, serum albumin, cholesterol, and complement. Rule out diabetes and SLE, as well as drug exposure, underlying malignancy, and infection. If no systemic disease or exposure can be discovered, then a renal biopsy is indicated.

RENAL FAILURE

BIG BUNS

Blood flow problem (pre-renal)
Intrinsic renal disease (renal)
GI/internal bleeding (metabolism of heme)

Bladder outlet obstruction (post-renal)
Ureteral/collecting system obstruction (post-renal)
Nephrotoxins (e.g., drugs, rhabdomyolysis, uric acid)
Steroids (catabolic states)

Notes

1. An elevated blood urea nitrogen (BUN) level may indicate renal insufficiency (reduced GFR) or may occur secondary to increased catabolism of proteins (e.g., steroid therapy) or with increased metabolism of heme products (e.g., GI or other internal bleeding). "BIG BUNS" provides a quick list of causes of a rising BUN. When renal insufficiency is the cause of a rising BUN, it is helpful to categorize etiologies as **pre-renal, renal,** or **post-renal**. Pre-renal azotemia occurs when renal blood is reduced and, as a consequence, renal filtration (GFR). Prerenal causes include volume depletion, heart failure, vascular disease, and shock. Renal

causes of low urine output result from damage or disease of the renal parenchyma, including the glomeruli, interstitium, and tubules. Toxins, vasculitides, interstitial diseases, and primary glomerulonephritides are among the causes. Post-renal conditions that lead to low urine output are characterized by an anatomic obstruction to urine output. The most common of these is prostate enlargement, although papillary necrosis, bilateral ureteral obstruction, and bladder outlet obstruction are possible causes. There is, of course, overlap in etiologies (e.g., CHF may precipitate ATN), but this classification is useful in organizing diagnostic possibilities.

2. The following mnemonic lists most of the causes of renal failure according to pre-renal, renal, and post-renal mechanisms:

I CHASE A RISING BUN

Pre-renal
Intravascular volume depletion (dehydration, third spacing)

Cardiac causes (CHF, MI, tamponade)
Hepatorenal syndrome
Arterial disease (renal artery stenosis)
Shock
Eclampsia/obstetrical complications

Pre-renal/Renal
Acute tubular necrosis

Renal
Radiographic contrast and other toxins (drugs, rhabdomyolysis, hemolysis)
Intrarenal emboli (cholesterol, DIC)
Scleroderma
Interstitial nephritis
Necrotizing vasculitis (polyarteritis, nodosa, Wegener's)
Glomerulonephritis

Post-renal
Bladder obstruction (usually prostatism, sometimes blood, pus, calculi)
Ureteral obstruction (calculi, retroperitoneal fibrosis, cancer)
Necrosis of renal papillae (diabetes, sickle cell anemia, NSAID abuse, infection)

3. The usual approach again depends on the history and physical evaluation. Frequently, prerenal causes are obvious, such as CHF and cirrhosis. Post-renal causes can be excluded in appropriate patients by placement of a Foley catheter. BUN and creatinine may further help to identify the pathogenesis. In pre-renal causes, BUN rises disproportionately to creatinine (often in a ratio of 20:1 or greater), while in renal causes, creatine elevation usually is more pronounced. Pre-existing renal disease may confound these parameters and is a common factor in low urine output.

4. When the etiology is still in question, a renal ultrasound is helpful to evaluate the collecting system for presence of obstruction and to assess renal size. Small, shrunken kidneys indicate long-standing disease that is unlikely to be reversible. Normal or large kidneys may be indicative of more acute disease. Certain serologic tests and renal biopsy may be appropriate. Prompt renal biopsy is especially important in cases of progressive renal insufficiency when immunosuppressive therapy may preserve renal function (e.g., vasculitis).

5. Hypocomplementemic renal failure: **"COMPS"**

    Cryoglobulinemia
    Occult infection (endocarditis, "shunt" nephritis)
    Membranoproliferative glomerulonephritis
    Post-streptococcal glomerulonephritis
    Systemic lupus erythematosus

Low complement levels are occasionally helpful in the differential diagnosis of glomerulonephritis, significantly narrowing the list of diagnostic possibilities. The role of complement in glomerular injury and progression of renal insufficiency is not clear. In idiopathic membranoproliferative glomerulonephritis, an antibody called C_3 nephritic factor is capable of inducing C_3 cleavage and probably causes the persistent depression of C_3 levels. This entity often is seen in association with hepatitis B infection.

RENAL STONES

OUCHS

Oxalate
Urate
Cystine
Hypercalcemia
Struvite

Notes

1. Kidney stones are among the most painful of afflictions, hence the mnemonic OUCHS.

2. **Oxalate** is a common component of kidney stones. Hyperoxaluria can occur in malabsorptive gastrointestinal disorders, such as Crohn's disease and ulcerative colitis. Normally, free oxalate is bound by calcium in the gut and is not absorbed. Malabsorbed fat binds calcium, leading to free luminal oxalate. Free oxalate is readily absorbed and then excreted in the urine. High levels of oxalate in the urine precipitate calcium oxalate stone formation.

3. **Uric** acid stones occur with low pH and supersaturation of the urine with undissociated uric acid. Myeloproliferative disease, chemotherapy, and Lesch-Nyhan syndrome cause massive production and excretion of uric acid. In gout, dehydration, and idiopathic uric acid lithiasis, urine pH is usually low. Uric acid facilitates heterogenous nucleation of calcium oxalate; thus, hyperuricosuria causes calcium oxalate stones.

4. **Cystine** stones are rare and are seen in patients with hereditary cystinosis.

5. **Hypercalcemia** (e.g., hyperparathyroidism, neoplastic hypercalcemia) increases urinary calcium concentration and precipitates calcium stone formation. Hypercalciuria may be idiopathic or result from renal tubular disease. In distal renal tubular acidosis, an alkaline urine and low urinary citrate levels favor formation of calcium phosphate stones.

6. **Struvite** stones ($MgNH_4PO_4$) occur mainly in women and result from urinary tract infections with urease-producing organisms (usually Proteus). Struvite stones may grow quite large and fill the renal pelvis ("staghorn calculus").

VIII

ACID-BASE

General Considerations

Arterial Blood Gas Interpretation

The interpretation of an arterial blood gas can be simplified by the steps outlined in the mnemonic **"ABG READ"**:

Accurate ABG? (Henderson-Hasselbalch)
Basic or acidic? (primary disorder)
Gap/delta gap (anion gap)

Respiratory or metabolic?
Extreme disturbance?
Appropriate compensation?
Double or triple disorder?

First, determine if the gas is **accurate** by determining the hydrogen ion concentration [H$^+$] using the Henderson-Hasselbalch equation:

$$[H^+] = 24 \times [pCO_2] / [HCO_3^-]$$

A simple way to recall this relationship is to remember that [H$^+$] increases as the pCO$_2$ increases or [HCO$_3^-$] decreases. The [H$^+$] for a given pH can be determined by either of the following methods: **(1)** Remember that at pH 7.2–7.5, every 0.1 unit change in pH changes [H$^+$] concentration by .10 mEq/L in the opposite direction. So, if [H$^+$] for pH 7.4 is 40 mEq/L, then [H$^+$] for pH 7.5 is 30 mEq/L and [H$^+$] for pH 7.3 is 50 mEq/L. **(2)** With every 0.1 unit rise in pH, multiply the preceding [H$^+$] by 0.8 (e.g., for a change in pH from 7.4 to 7.5, 40 mEq/L × 0.8 = 32 mEq/L). Conversely, for every 0.1 unit fall in pH, multiply the preceding [H$^+$] by 1.25 (e.g., for a change in pH from 7.4 to 7.3, 40 mEq/L × 1.25 = 50).

The second method is slightly more accurate, but either method is usually sufficient for confirming accuracy. The following lists the [H$^+$] for a given pH:

pH 7.8, [H+] = 16.4
pH 7.7, [H+] = 20.5
pH 7.6, [H+] = 25.6
pH 7.5, [H+] = 32
pH 7.4, [H+] = 40
pH 7.3, [H+] = 50
pH 7.2, [H+] = 62.5
pH 7.1, [H+] = 78.5
pH 7.0, [H+] = 97.7
pH 6.9, [H+] = 122.1

The components of the bicarbonate/carbonic acid system are always in equilibrium in the blood, and so pH, pCO_2, and [HCO_3^-] measured by venous blood chemistry should adhere to the constraints of Henderson-Hasselbalch. If there is disagreement, then a laboratory or collection error has occurred and repeat determination should be obtained.

To assess the accuracy of oxygenation, add the pO_2 and pCO_2. If the total is greater than 140 TORR (at sea level), then the patient was on supplemental oxygen or a laboratory error was made. The oxygen level decreases with age, which can be estimated by subtracting 1 TORR from 80 for every year of age above 60. So, an 80-year-old patient should have a pO_2 no less than 60 at sea level.

After establishing the consistency of the values for pH, pCO_2, and [HCO_3^-], look at the pH to establish if the primary or dominant disorder is **basic or acidic**. Since there is no over-compensation for an acid-base disorder, the primary disturbance is determined by the pH. Occasionally, a chronic respiratory acidosis or alkalosis may have a normal pH in the absence of a mixed disorder.

Next, the **serum anion gap**, $[Na^+] - ([Cl^-] + HCO_3^-)$, is calculated to look for the presence of unmeasured anions, as occurs with the addition of any strong acid to body fluids. The anion gap can be altered in the absence of an acid-base disorder. A low serum albumin or an increase in unmeasured cation, such as occurs with lithium ingestion or when certain paraproteins are present in multiple myeloma, may decrease the gap (see Low Anion Gap section). On the other hand, metabolic alkalosis may modestly increase the anion gap. An increase in the anion gap usually indicates the presence of a metabolic acidosis, but the normal anion gap varies widely, with an average value of 10–12 mEq/L. Given the large number of factors that can affect the anion gap, previous electrolytes measurements from the patient may be helpful for comparison.

With a high anion gap metabolic acidosis, there should be a close reciprocal relationship between the rise in anion gap and the decrease of serum [HCO_3^-], called the **delta gap**. The delta gap is defined as (anion gap − 12). In simple gap acidosis, a reduction in serum [HCO_3^-] by 10 is associated with an increase in anion gap of 10. Addition of the value for delta gap to the measured [HCO_3^-] allows you to determine the [HCO_3^-] level that existed prior to the development of the gap acidosis. Thus, if delta gap + [HCO_3^-] is in the normal range for serum [HCO_3^-], then a simple anion gap acidosis is present (i.e., the added acid has caused the expected drop in [HCO_3^-]). If the value is outside the normal range, then another disorder must have been present prior to the development of the gap acidosis.

The following rules summarize the use of delta gap after a high anion gap is detected:

$28 \geq$ delta gap + [HCO_3^-] ≥ 23, simple high gap acidosis

Delta gap + [HCO_3^-] < 23, a non-anion gap acidosis also is present.

Delta gap + [HCO_3^-] ≥ 28, a metabolic alkalosis also is present.

Next, determine the specific type of acidic or basic disorder. Acid-base disorders can be classified as either **respiratory or metabolic**. Respiratory disorders are initiated by a change in $PaCO_2$ while metabolic disorders are initiated by a change in [HCO_3^-]. These primary disturbances initiate predictable compensatory changes (see below).

Look to see if there is an extreme change in pH, pCO_2, or [HCO_3^-], as this often indicates an acute process or two processes that cause the pH to change in the same direction (e.g., a metabolic alkalosis and respiratory alkalosis as occurs in a pregnant patient who has severe vomiting from hyperemesis gravida, or COPD with CO_2 retention and hypoxia causing lactic acidosis). Acid-base disturbances in which the response to a primary disturbance is obviously inappropriate (e.g., increase pCO_2 with metabolic acidosis) are mixed and do not require the use of predictive formulas. Extreme disturbances require rapid therapy.

If the changes in pH, pCO_2, and [HCO_3^-] are not extreme and do not represent an inappropriate direction of compensation, then assess whether **appropriate compensation** has occurred by using specific predictive formulae. These formulae are useful in predicting the appropriate degree of response, but keep in mind that an appropriate ventilatory response for a metabolic disturbance may take 12 hours to occur, and adequate renal compensation for a respiratory disorder may take several days to occur. It is also important to understand that the compensatory responses do not normalize the pH. Exception: occasionally, chronic respiratory acidosis or alkalosis may have a normal pH.

Summary of the Primary Disturbances and Compensatory Responses for Acid-Base Disorders

Disorder	Primary Disturbance	Compen-satory Response	Type	Appropriate Response for a Single Disorder	Comments
Respiratory acidosis	Increased pCO_2	Increased HCO_3	Acute	For each change in pCO_2 of 10 TORR (from normal pCO_2 of 40 TORR), expected change	pH is lower than chronic acidosis Uncomplicated acute respiratory acidosis

Table continued on next page.

Summary of the Primary Disturbances and Compensatory Responses for Acid-Base Disorders (Continued)

Disorder	Primary Disturbance	Compensatory Response	Type	Appropriate Response for a Single Disorder	
Respiratory acidosis (cont.)	Increased pCO_2 (cont.)	Increased HCO_3 (cont.)	Acute (cont.)	in pH is 0.08 units (patient with pCO_2 of 60 should have pH of 20/10 × 0.08 = 0.16, so predicted pH is 7.4 − 0.16 = 7.24). HCO_3 increases 1 mmol/L for each 10 mmHg increase in pCO_2	will not elevate [HCO_3^-] over 32 unless superimposed metabolic alkalosis is present
			Chronic	For each change in pCO_2 of 10 TORR from normal pCO_2 of 40 TORR, expected change in pH is 0.03 units (patient with pCO_2 of 60 should have pH of 20/10 × 0.03 = 0.06, so predicted pH is 7.4 − 0.06 = 7.34). HCO_3 increases 3–3.5 mmol/L for each 10 mmHg increase in pCO_2.	pH less than normal, but may be normal. Unusual for patients with $pCO_2 > 60$ TORR to have normal pH.
Respiratory alkalosis	Decreased pCO_2	Decreased HCO_3	Acute	Same rule as acute respiratory acidosis (patient with pCO_2 of 20 should have pH of 7.56). HCO_3 decreases 2 mmol/L for each 10 mmHg decrease in pCO_2.	pH is higher than chronic alkalosis
			Chronic	Same rule as chronic respiratory acidosis (patient with pCO_2 of 20 should have pH of 7.46).	Unusual for HCO_3^- to fall to less than 15 mEq/L in absence of

Table continued on next page.

Disorder	Primary Disturbance	Compen-satory Response	Type	Appropriate Response for a Single Disorder	
Respiratory alkalosis *(cont.)*	Decreased pCO_2 *(cont.)*	Decreased HCO_3 *(cont.)*	Chronic *(cont.)*	HCO_3 decreases 4–5 mmol/L for each 10 mmHg decrease in pCO_2.	accompanying metabolic acidosis. The pH is often normal.
Metabolic acidosis	Decreased HCO_3	Decreased pCO_2	—	$pCO_2 = [1.5(HCO_3) + 8] \pm 2$ (patient with metabolic acidosis and HCO_3 of 10 should have pCO_2 of $[1.5(10) + 8] \pm 2 = 23 \pm 2 = 21{-}25$ TORR. $pCO_2 =$ last 2 digits of pH × 100.	Full compensation (hyperventilation) may take 12–24 hours
Metabolic alkalosis	Increased HCO_3	Increased pCO_2	—	$pCO_2 = 0.9^*$ $(HCO_3) + 9$ (patient with metabolic alkalosis and HCO_3 of 40 should have pCO_2 of $0.9^* (40) + 9 = 45$ TORR). * range = 0.6–0.9	Compensation less consistent than for metabolic acidosis. $pCO_2 > 45$ occurs in 25% of cases. Rare to see $pCO_2 > 55$ TORR except in severe alkalosis or superimposed respiratory alkalosis.

After checking for appropriate compensation, decide if the disorder is simple or if a **double or triple** disturbance is present. Types of mixed disorders and clues to their presence are as follows:

1. **Metabolic alkalosis + respiratory alkalosis**—Both processes increase the pH. A decreased pCO_2 is seen with increased HCO_3. A very high pH is possible because the alkaloses summate. There is a mild elevation of anion gap. Hypokalemia frequently is present. Example: pregnancy with vomiting.

2. **Respiratory acidosis + metabolic alkalosis**—Both processes increase the HCO_3. Often there is a normal pH and a very high HCO_3. pCO_2 is higher than predicted on the basis of metabolic alkalosis alone. Example: COPD + diuretic therapy.

3. **Metabolic acidosis + respiratory acidosis**—Both processes decrease the pH. pH is very low because the acidoses summate. Example: decompensated COPD + lactic acidosis.

4. **Metabolic acidosis + metabolic alkalosis**—The two processes change the HCO_3 and the pCO_2 in opposite directions. The pH may be increased, decreased, or normal, depending on the relative severity of the two processes. Consider this diagnosis when the anion gap is increased, but the HCO_3 is not decreased. Example: DKA + vomiting.

5. **Metabolic acidosis + respiratory alkalosis**—Both processes decrease the HCO_3. Consider this diagnosis when a metabolic acidosis is accompanied by a pCO_2 that is lower than predicted, or when respiratory alkalosis is associated with an HCO_3 measurement lower than predicted. Example: salicylate overdose.

6. **Triple acid-base disturbance**—triple disturbances occur when a mixed metabolic acidosis + metabolic alkalosis is complicated by either a respiratory acidosis or a respiratory alkalosis. While mixtures of metabolic disturbances may occur, mixed respiratory disturbances cannot occur by definition, because a person can never concurrently over- and under-excrete CO_2. The diagnosis of a triple disturbance is generally made in a patient with metabolic alkalosis and respiratory acidosis or alkalosis in whom the anion gap is found to be significantly increased (> 16). Example: DKA + vomiting + obtundation/hypoventilation.

Clinical Conditions and Diagnoses

METABOLIC ACIDOSIS WITH A HIGH ANION GAP

KLUES

Ketoacidoses
Lactic acidoses
Uremia (organic acids)
Ethylene glycol and the alcohols
Salicylates

Notes

1. This mnemonic lists the primary conditions in which the anion gap, $\{[Na^+] - ([Cl] + [HCO_3])]\}$, increases. Because of **electroneutrality**, unmeasured anions must increase as bicarbonate falls, leading to a widening of the anion gap. "KLUES" to the cause of an increased anion gap come from the history and laboratory tests, including BUN, creatinine, glucose, lactate, serum ketones, serum osmolality, and a toxin screen.

2. **Ketoacidosis** occurs in three settings: **diabetes, alcoholism,** and **malnutrition ("DAM!").** In diabetic ketoacidosis, acetoacetic and beta-hydroxybutyric acids are produced more rapidly than they can be metabolized. They accumulate, causing a drop in plasma bicarbonate and a rise in the anion gap. Alcoholics may have poor food intake and vomiting associated with high ethanol intake, causing ketoacidosis and an elevated anion gap. The ketoacidosis may be missed because the nitroprusside test for ketones only detects acetoacetic acid and not beta-hydroxybutyric acid, which tends to predominate. Malnutrition alone may cause a modest ketoacidosis. Reduced carbohydrate levels cause low insulin and high glucagon. These hormonal changes (also relevant to DKA and alcoholic ketosis) favor glycolysis and ketogenesis.

3. **Uremia** is characterized by the accumulation of **organic acids**, which normally are excreted by the kidney. In acute renal failure, plasma bicarbonate falls by 1 to 2 mmol/L per day if impaired renal acid excretion is the sole cause of metabolic acidosis. Greater rates of decline suggest the presence of an additional cause of acid production. In chronic renal failure, the bicarbonate tends to stabilize at levels of 12–18 mmol/L and rarely falls below 10 mmol/L unless another disorder is present.

4. **Lactic acidosis** occurs when there is an imbalance between lactate production and elimination **("LACTIC")**. During anaerobic conditions, glycolysis is accelerated and pyruvate increases. Pyruvate is in equilibrium with lactate; thus, lactate levels increase. Since one proton is generated for each lactate molecule produced, acidosis is the result of lactate production.

Because the liver is the major organ for metabolizing lactate, severe **liver disease** causes lactic acidosis. Lactate production is normal, but metabolism is impaired. With significant liver dysfunction, the normal lactate load produced by the body is not metabolized, lactate accumulates, and acidosis ensues.

Selective dysfunction of mitochondria (e.g., congenital disease, biguanide toxicity) causes lactic acidosis in the absence of other evidence of liver dysfunction. Lactate overproduction results from circulatory failure. Tissue hypoxia, as occurs with **cardiopulmonary arrest, carbon monoxide** poisoning and severe anemia, leads to lactic acidosis. Vigorous exercise or muscular **tetany** as occurs with seizures may cause a transient rise in lactate. Systemic **infection/sepsis** causes circulatory shock, organ hypoperfusion, and subsequent lactate production. Lactic acidosis may complicate **cancers**, such as leukemia and lymphoma, when tissue hypoxia is not in evidence. Overproduction of lactate by the malignant tissue may be a factor.

Note that lactic acidosis also may contribute to the severe acidosis seen with salicylate, methanol, or ethylene glycol poisonings.

5. **Ethylene glycol** and **methanol** are converted to acidic metabolites, which accumulate in the blood. An increase in osmolar gap is characteristic, and prompt intervention is critical. Isopropyl alcohol causes a more modest increase in anion gap and serum osmolality.

6. **Salicylates** cause a characteristic initial respiratory alkalosis by stimulating central respiration. The presence of respiratory alkalosis combined with an increased anion gap frequently occurs with salicylate intoxication and should not be missed.

7. Certain gastrointestinal disorders have been reported to cause a gap acidosis secondary to accumulation of **D-lactate**. It is thought that certain bacteria produce D-lactate in the gut that is systemically absorbed. A special serum assay for D-lactate is available, as it is not detected by the conventional assay.

8. Other drugs have been associated with a gap acidosis. Isoniazid causes refractory seizures and a subsequent lactic acidosis. Paraldehyde is rarely used, and its role in causing gap acidosis is not well documented, but it is remembered because of the familiar **"MUD PILES"** mnemonic (methanol, uremia, DKA, paraldehyde, isopropyl alcohol, lactic acid, ethylene glycol, salicylates). **Propylene glycol**, a diluent used in some intravenous medications (e.g., nitroglycerine), may rarely cause a secondary lactic acidosis.

9. When measured plasma osmolality exceeds the calculated osmolality **[(2 × plasma Na) + glucose/18 + BUN/2.8]**, suspect ethylene glycol or methanol toxicity. Ethanol intoxication and some cases of lactic acidosis or alcoholic ketosis also may feature a small "osmolal gap" (up to 10–15 mOsm/kg).

DAM U LACTIC GAPS

Ketoacidoses
Diabetic ketoacidoses
Alcoholic ketosis
Malnutrition

Organic acids
Uremia

Lactic acidoses
Liver disease
Arrest
Carbon monoxide poisoning
Tetany/seizures (rhabdomyolysis)
Infection/sepsis
Cancer

Other unmeasured anions
Gastrointestinal disease (D-lactate)
Alcohols/anti-freeze
Propylene glycol/paraldehyde
Salicylates

METABOLIC ACIDOSES WITH A NORMAL ANION GAP

GUT

Gastrointestinal losses (diarrhea, pancreatic fistula)
Urinary losses
Total parenteral nutrition

Notes

1. Normal anion gap or hyperchloremic acidoses almost always result from HCO_3 loss from the GI tract or from the kidney. As the above mnemonic suggests, GUT losses from diarrhea are the most common cause. Urinary losses from renal tubular disease are less common.

2. In both GI and renal disorders, sodium bicarbonate stores are low, and sodium chloride is retained in excessive amounts to preserve volume status. The urine net charge or **urinary anion gap**, { ([Na]+[K] – [Cl] }, is useful in differentiating between renal and gastrointestinal causes of HCO_3 loss. Urinary acidification results from the excretion of ammonium, NH_4^+. The presence of the positive ion, NH_4^+, indicates that other major cations, **[Na]+[K]**, are present in lower amounts when compared to the major anion, **[CL]**. A negative urine anion gap implies the presence of NH_4^+ in the urine, indicating appropriate renal acidification in response to acidosis (as in GI losses). A positive value indicates a renal acidification defect (no NH_4^+ in the urine). If the cause appears to be renal dysfunction (positive urinary anion gap), then the serum potassium is helpful. Low potassium suggests an H^+ secretion defect, whereas high values are consistent with deficient aldosterone action (Type IV renal tubular acidosis [RTA]).

3. In rare cases, iatrogenic normal gap acidosis results from intravenous administration of TPN or acidic amino acid solutions, ammonium chloride or hydrochloric acid. An apparent, normal gap acidosis is occasionally seen when a gap acidosis is accompanied by a pre-existing condition that lowers the anion gap, such as hypoalbuminemia or a cationic paraprotein (see Low Anion Gap section).

4. **Respiratory alkalosis** with reduced pCO_2 levels leads to a loss of bicarbonate. With **rapid correction** (i.e., decreased respiratory rate), pCO_2 returns to normal, but bicarbonate conservation and reclamation by the kidney takes 24 to 48 hours to return levels to normal. A transient non-gap acidosis occurs.

5. In **DKA**, it is common to see an incidental hyperchloremic acidosis in the **recovery** phase. This phenomenon occurs because sodium chloride is retained with volume repletion. The ketones (a source for regenerating bicarbonate) are lost in the urine, and bicarbonate regeneration is slowed. Similarly, vigorous volume replacement in a dehydrated patient suppresses aldosterone secretion. Since aldosterone increases bicarbonate regeneration and absorption, the lower levels tend to maintain the hyperchloremic state. This "expansion acidosis" is the converse of the "contraction alkalosis" seen with volume depletion; the latter is a high aldosterone state. The acidosis from volume replacement is rarely of clinical significance.

6. A more comprehensive listing of causes of non-gap acidoses is listed below. The mnemonic emphasizes the importance of calculating the urine gap when the cause is uncertain.

URINE GAP: NA+K–CL

Ureterosigmoidostomy
RTA
Intestinal disease (diarrhea)
NH$_4^+$/TPN
Early renal failure

Glue sniffing (toluene)
Aldosterone deficiency
Pancreatic fistula

NaCl infusion ("expansion" acidosis)
After DKA or respiratory alkalosis

K$^+$-sparing diuretics

Carbonic anhydrase inhibitors (impairs urine acidification)
Laxative abuse (GI losses)

Low Anion Gap

ALBUMIN

Albumin loss
Lithium
Bromine
Unmeasured cations (K, Mg, Ca)
Myeloma (cationic paraprotein)
Iodide
Na$^+$ underestimation/artifact

Notes

1. A low serum **albumin** is the most common cause of low anion gap. The normal anion gap is approximately 5–12. Because of this wide range of normal and the many factors affecting the anion gap, the clinical usefulness of a low measured anion gap has been questioned. Knowing the factors that affect the anion gap is perhaps most useful when trying to determine the significance of modest changes in the anion gap (e.g., an anion gap of 16 may be significant in a patient with a very low albumin). A reduction in the anion gap may also be due to laboratory error.

2. A lower serum anion gap may be observed in conditions with an increase in **unmeasured cations**, such as occurs with hyperkalemia, hypercalcemia, or hypermagnesemia. It may also be seen when there is an increase in unmeasured cations that are not normally present, such as with **multiple myeloma**, polyclonal gammopathy, or **lithium**. A low gap is seen with a decrease in unmeasured anions (usually hypoalbuminemia). **Sodium underestimation** is much less likely to occur given new direct ion-selective techniques (a low gap was more common previously in cases of hyperviscosity and severe hypernatremia). Chloride overestimation was formally seen in cases of hypertriglyceridemia, but this also is less of a problem now. However, **bromine** and **iodide** may lead to chloride overestimation and thus reduce the anion gap. Bromine and iodide have slightly lower renal clearances than chloride. Electrolyte measurements do not distinguish between bromine or iodide and chloride, so a rise in bromine or iodide is falsely measured as an ever greater rise in chloride. Other rarely reported causes of a low serum anion gap include renal transplantation and hyponatremia.

3. Clearly, there are many considerations in calculating the anion gap—particularly in a patient with multiple medical problems. Take all of these factors into account when interpreting the anion gap.

METABOLIC ALKALOSIS

ALDOS

Aldosterone
Lasix
Dehydration
Over-ventilation
Stomach losses

Notes

1. Metabolic alkalosis is not a specific disease; it is usually a response to NaCl and K$^+$ deficit. Understanding the hormone aldosterone is the key to understanding most cases of metabolic alkalosis; hence, the mnemonic ALDOS. Aldosterone promotes renal acidification and concomitant bicarbonate regeneration and absorption. Primary hyperaldosteronism and other hypermineralocorticoid states cause metabolic alkalosis. Similarly, volume depletion causes a secondary increase in aldosterone, also promoting metabolic alkalosis. With volume contraction, there is an increase in sodium avidity due to aldosterone activity. Because of electroneutrality, anions must be reabsorbed with sodium; therefore, chloride is maximally reabsorbed, leaving very little chloride in the urine. For this reason, the measurement of urine chloride (see mnemonic next page) is helpful in determining the cause of metabolic alkalosis.

2. The majority of metabolic alkalosis cases are due to extracellular fluid volume contraction and respond to saline administration. These so-called **saline-sensitive** types commonly result from vomiting and diuretic use. In these instances, volume loss leads to renal sodium conservation, necessitating maximal reabsorption of chloride as an obligate anion. Urine chloride is usually less than 10 mmoles/L in saline-sensitive metabolic alkalosis. Replacement of the volume deficit corrects the alkalosis.

3. Hypermineralocorticoidism (primary, Cushing's syndrome, renal artery stenosis, malignant hypertension, J-G cell tumor, Bartter's syndrome, and licorice gluttony) is the other major mechanism that can maintain metabolic alkalosis. These conditions are **saline-sensitive** and typically have a urine chloride concentration > 20 mmoles/L. The patient's volume status helps to differentiate between a saline-sensitive cause (low volume) and a saline-insensitive cause (normal or increased volume). Rarely, patients with extracellular fluid volume depletion have other causes for metabolic alkalosis (magnesium depletion, Bartter's syndrome). Liddle's syndrome is a rare disorder in which patients appear to have hyperaldosteronism,

but aldosterone levels are low. It is probably due to an intrinsic tubular defect and can be treated with traimterene or amiloride, but not spironolactone.

4. The following mnemonic lists the specific causes of metabolic alkalosis:

RENAL CL⁻ EVAL

Recovery from hypercapnia, organic acidosis
Emesis
Nasogastric suction
Aldosteronism
Lasix/loop diuretics

Cystic fibrosis
Low K^+, Mg^{++}

Exsanguination/massive transfusion (citrate)
Volume depletion
Alkalai intake (IV bicarb, milk-alkalai)
Liddle's syndrome

RESPIRATORY ACIDOSIS

COPDS

Cardiac arrest
Obtundation
Pulmonary disease/airway obstruction
Drugs/overdose
Skeletal/neuromuscular disease

Notes

1. Respiratory acidosis represents a failure of ventilation. Obstructive lung disease is the most common cause of both acute and chronic respiratory acidosis, hence the mnemonic COPDS.

2. Common causes of hypoventilation and subsequent respiratory acidosis include cardiac arrest, obtundation, pulmonary disease or large airway obstruction, CNS-depressing drugs/overdose, and skeletal/neuromuscular disease (e.g., ALS, myasthenia gravis, advanced kyphoscoliosis).

RESPIRATORY ALKALOSIS

PCO$_2$ VENTS

Pregnancy   **V**entilator
Cirrhosis   **E**mbolus
O$_2$ deficit   **N**eurologic disease
                        Temperature (fever, heat)
                        Salicylates/drugs

N otes

1. In contrast to respiratory acidosis, respiratory alkalosis is secondary to hyperventilation. Over-excretion of carbon dioxide, PCO$_2$ VENTS, accounts for the alkalosis.
2. Respiratory center stimulation in **pregnancy** is due to increased production of progesterone, while in **cirrhosis** there probably is decreased metabolism of substances that stimulate the respiratory center. Hypoxia (**O$_2$ deficit**) also causes hyperventilation. Patients on mechanical **ventilators** may have respiratory alkalosis when the minute ventilation is inappropriately high. Tachypnea and respiratory alkalosis is a very sensitive albeit nonspecific sign of pulmonary **embolus**. CNS injury or **neurologic diseases** also may cause hyperventilation. **Temperature** elevations with fever or heat exhaustion stimulate breathing, and respiratory alkalosis is the initial acid-base abnormality in **salicylate overdose**.

IX

GASTROENTEROLOGY

Clinical Symptoms and Signs

ABDOMINAL PAIN

MEAN GUT

Metabolic
Endocrine
Abdominal
Neurogenic

Gynecologic/genitalia
Urinary/renal system
Thoracic

Notes

1. "MEAN GUT" provides a simple outline for approaching abdominal pain. The most important initial decision is whether urgent surgical intervention or diagnostic testing is indicated. The history and physical examination and a few simple tests guide the decision-making. It is essential to exclude extra-abdominal causes of pain (i.e., metabolic, endocrinologic, neurologic, gynecologic, urologic, and thoracic) before embarking on expensive and invasive testing.

2. **Metabolic** causes of abdominal pain include uremia, porphyria, C1 esterase deficiency, Familial Mediterranean Fever, and poisons (e.g., heavy metals, envenomation, chemotherapy). **Endocrine** causes include adrenal insufficiency, hypercalcemia, and diabetic ketoacidosis. Most of the intra-**abdominal** etiologies

of pain are listed in the "PREP FOR SURGICAL APPENDECTOMY?" mnemonic on page 172. **Neurogenic** causes of pain include herpes zoster, tabes dorsalis, psychogenic pain, functional bowel disease, and spinal radiculitis. **Gynecologic** causes of pain—important in any female patient and especially those of menstruating age—and **urologic** causes of pain, such as renal stones, pyelonephritis, and urinary retention, also are included in the differential for appendicitis. Finally, pain may be referred from **thoracic** problems such as pneumonia and myocardial ischemia. Esophageal disease usually causes chest discomfort, although patients may complain of abdominal symptoms.

3. The initial diagnostic evaluation of a patient with acute abdominal pain often includes CBC, urinalysis, amylase and/or lipase, liver enzymes, and abdominal x-rays, taken with the patient in the upright position to evaluate for dilated loops of bowel or free air. Other tests may be appropriate in selected patients, such as serum electrolytes, BUN, creatinine, calcium, cosyntropin stimulation testing for adrenal insufficiency, or a chest radiograph.

4. Important tips for internists:

   a. Be careful to exclude metabolic derangements, systemic diseases and extra-abdominal processes, which may present with abdominal pain.

   b. Rule out ectopic pregnancy in any female of menstruating age. Pelvic examination should be performed on virtually all women with acute abdominal pain. Every woman of reproductive age must have a pregnancy test.

   c. Elderly patients with acute abdominal processes may have atypical presentations and should be managed with greater caution. Mesenteric ischemia, for example, may present with severe pain and an unimpressive physical examination (i.e., pain out of proportion to the clinical findings). Also, patients on corticosteroid therapy may have atypical presentations, as steroids may mask clinical findings.

5. The location, duration, progression, and onset of pain (see table) can be helpful in differentiating between causes of abdominal pain. There is considerable overlap, but a general time course is often helpful in discerning the cause of abdominal pain. Relieving and aggravating factors are helpful in localizing the source. For example, pain relieved by the passage of bowel movements suggests the colon as a likely source. Pain initiated by swallowing implicates the esophagus, while pain aggravated by any action that moves the abdomen suggests peritonitis (the patient usually prefers to lie still). On the other hand, with obstruction of a hollow viscus, patients usually move about in an attempt to seek relief, and movement does not make the pain worse.

Pain According to the Acuity of Onset

Abrupt-Onset Pain (instant)

Gastrointestinal Causes	*Nongastrointestinal Causes*
Perforated ulcer	Ruptured or dissecting aneurysm
Ruptured abscess or hematoma	Ruptured ectopic pregnancy
Intestinal infarct	Pneumothorax
Ruptured esophagus	Myocardial infarction
	Pulmonary infarction
	Dissecting aneurysm

Rapid-Onset Pain (minutes)

Gastrointestinal Causes	*Nongastrointestinal Causes*
Perforated viscus	Ureteral colic
Strangulated viscus	Renal colic
Volvulus	Ectopic pregnancy
Pancreatitis	
Biliary colic	
Mesenteric infarct	
Diverticulitis	
Penetrating peptic ulcer	
High intestinal obstruction	
Appendicitis (gradual onset more common)	

Gradual-Onset Pain (hours)

Gastrointestinal Causes	*Nongastrointestinal Causes*
Appendicitis	Cystitis
Strangulated hernia	Pyelitis
Low intestinal obstruction	Salpingitis
Cholecystitis	Prostatitis
Pancreatitis	Threatened abortion
Gastritis	Urinary retention
Peptic ulcer	Pneumonitis
Colonic diverticulitis	
Meckel's diverticulitis	
Crohn's disease	
Ulcerative colitis	
Mesenteric lymphadenitis	
Abscess	
Intestinal infarct	
Mesenteric cyst	

6. Here is a mnemonic delineating the differential diagnosis for appendicitis:

PREP FOR SURGICAL APPENDECTOMY?

Pyelonephritis
Renal stone
Ectopic pregnancy
Pelvic inflammatory disease

Follicle rupture (mittelschmerz)
Ovarian cyst torsion
Rupture of corpus luteal cyst

Splenic rupture
Urinary retention
Ruptured aneurysm
Gastroenteritis
Infarcted/ischemic gut
Crohn's/ulcerative colitis
Abscess
Liver capsule distension/irritation

Appendicitis
Pancreatitis
Perforated ulcer
Esophageal rupture
No disease
Diverticulitis
Endometriosis
Cholecystitis
Twisted bowel
Obstructed bowel
Meckel's diverticulum
Yersinia/lymphadenitis

DIARRHEA

SOILING

Secretory
Osmotic
Inflammatory
Laxatives (factitious)
Ischemic
Neurogenic
Gastrointestinal bleeding

Notes

1. The primary mechanisms of diarrhea (or apparent diarrhea) are summarized by the mnemonic SOILING. Diarrhea is defined as an increase in daily stool weight above 200 grams per day. Since this is not a very easily obtained measure, diarrhea is here defined from the patient's perspective: an increase in stool frequency and/or liquidity. This definition includes hyperdefecation, which is an increase in frequency without an increase in stool weight as occurs in irritable bowel syndrome, hyperthyroidism, and fecal incontinence. Also included is gastrointestinal bleeding causing melena, which patients may describe as diarrhea.
2. **Secretory** (watery) diarrhea is characterized by voluminous fecal output not necessarily related to food intake, which fails to improve with fasting. There is perturbation of normal fluid and electrolyte transport in the gut, and the result is watery stools with normal electrolyte concentrations and no increase in stool osmolality. The classic examples of secretory diarrheas are hormonal, including carcinoid syndrome, Zollinger-Ellison, VIPoma, medullary thyroid carcinoma, and systemic mastocytosis. An exception is somatistatinoma, in which the diarrhea is osmotic with steatorrhea secondary to inhibition of pancreatic secretions and gall bladder motility. Bile salts stimulate colonic secretion, and processes that increase bile salt delivery to the colon also cause secretory diarrhea. Examples include: ileal bypass or resection (reduced reabsorption), truncal vagotomy (abnormal transit), and after cholecystectomy (reduced storage capacity).
3. **Osmotic** diarrheas (such as pancreatitis, sprue, bacterial overgrowth, and Whipple's disease) are characterized by bulky, greasy, foul-smelling stools, weight loss, and improvement in diarrhea with fasting. This form of diarrhea results from an ingested solute that is not absorbed by the small intestine. The unabsorbed solute exerts an osmotic force and draws fluid into the intestinal lumen. The resultant increased stool volume exceeds the colon's reabsorptive capacity,

and diarrhea ensues. Stool analysis shows a gap between electrolyte concentrations and total stool osmolality due to the unabsorbed solute.

4. Inflammatory causes (inflammatory bowel disease, radiation enterocolitis, eosinophilic gastroentereitis and certain AIDS-associated infections) are characterized by fever, abdominal pain, and blood and/or leukocytes in the stool. In these disorders there is inflammation and injury to the intestinal mucosa. The mechanism of diarrhea may include malabsorption or secretion due to disruption of normal mucosal functions.

5. Factitious diarrhea from **laxative abuse** is osmotic and should be suspected in women with chronic diarrhea, hypokalemia, and a history of psychiatric illness. Certain prescribed medications also can cause diarrhea, such as antacids, theophylline, colchicine, digitalis, and antibiotics.

6. Ischemia is *not* a common cause of diarrhea, and the clinical picture depends on the degree of vascular compromise. Acute, fulminant ischemic colitis is due to complete vessel occlusion and features severe abdominal pain, bloody diarrhea, and rapid decompensation. Nonocclusive ischemia has a less severe course and usually resolves without intervention. Patients with nonocclusive ischemia have lesser degrees of pain and bleeding, occurring over a longer period of time. Anorexia, vomiting, and diarrhea may be the primary complaints.

7. Neurogenic disorders are disturbances of intestinal motility that often cause hyperdefecation or incontinence as opposed to true diarrhea. The irritable bowel syndrome (IBS) is a common and increasingly recognized form of neurogenic diarrhea. IBS is characterized by alternating constipation and diarrhea, as well as diffuse abdominal pain. IBS begins by early adulthood and should not be accepted as a diagnosis in an older patient with recent-onset diarrhea. Other neurologic diseases (diabetes, cauda-equina syndrome, Shy-Drager) also can cause altered intestinal motility and diarrhea.

8. Gastrointestinal bleeding, when subacute, may cause frequent loose, black stools. Although not strictly diarrhea, patients may interpret it as such. Also, some of the other mechanisms of diarrhea may feature bleeding, especially the inflammatory etiologies and ischemia.

9. The majority of cases of **acute diarrhea** (< 7–14 days in duration) are infectious, the diagnosis of which can be suspected by a history of recent travel, ingestion of unusual food (raw seafood or undercooked poultry products or hamburger), or recent contact with people who have been sick. Infections by invasive bacteria (*Campylobacter, Shigella, Salmonella, Aeromonas,* certain *Escherichia coli*) are often associated with bloody diarrhea. It is important to exclude other causes of bloody diarrhea such as mesenteric ischemia and inflammatory bowel disease. Infections by noninvasive bacteria and protozoa (*Vibrio cholerae*, enterotoxigenic *E. coli, Klebsiella,* Giardia, Cryptosporidia) typically produce watery diarrhea without blood. *C. difficile* rarely causes bloody diarrhea. *Yersinia*, which commonly infects the terminal ileum and cecum, often presents with watery diarrhea and right lower quadrant pain, which can mimic appendicitis and Crohn's disease.

10. A more comprehensive list of the causes of **chronic diarrhea**, organized pathophysiologically, follows:

I RACE TO PASS LOTS OF WILD BM, FIND A CURE!

Ischemia
Ischemia

Secretory
Rectal villous adenoma
After cholecystectomy (cholerrheic)
Collagenous colitis (lymphocytic or microscopic colitis)
Endocrine (Zollinger-Ellison, VIPoma, carcinoid, medullary thyroid carcinoma, mastocytosis)

Truncal vagotomy
Obesity surgery (ileal bypass or resection)

Osmotic
Pancreatitis (chronic pancreatitis with steatorrhea)
Abetalipoproteinemia
Somatostatinoma
Short-bowel syndrome

Lymphangiectasia
Overgrowth of bacteria
Tropical sprue
Sprue (gluten-sensitive)

Olestra/dietetic foods
Fruits/candy (fructose, sorbital)

Whipple's disease
Infections causing steatorrhea (Isospora, Giardia, Strongyloides)
Lactose intolerance
Drugs causing steatorrhea (e.g., colchicine, neomycin)

Factitious or "pseudo" diarrhea
Bleeding (melena)
Münchausen's/malingering (laxative abuse)

Neurogenic or altered motility
Fecal incontinence or impaction (obstipation)
Irritable bowel
Neurologic diseases (e.g., autonomic neuropathies, cauda equina syndrome)
Diabetes mellitus

Inflammatory
AIDS-associated infections (chronic infections)

Crohn's disease
Ulcerative colitis
Radiation enterocolitis
Eosinophilic gastroenteritis

DYSPHAGIA

BITES

Blocked esophageal lumen
Intrinsic narrowing of the esophagus
Throat/mouth disease (oropharyngeal dysphagia)
Extrinsic compression of the esophagus
Smooth/**S**triated muscle disorders

N otes

1. There are five primary mechanisms of dysphagia. **Blockage of the esophageal lumen** results from impacted foreign bodies and swallowing too large a food bolus. Processes that cause **intrinsic narrowing of the esophagus** include herpes virus and other opportunistic infections, esophageal webs and rings, peptic strictures and caustic burns, benign and malignant tumors, and Crohn's disease. Abnormalities of the **throat and mouth** cause oropharyngeal dysphagia and include pharyngeal weakness from stroke, lack of saliva from Sjögren's syndrome and lesions affecting the tongue. **Extrinsic compression of the esophagus** may be caused by a thyroid mass, Zenker's diverticulum, vascular anomalies, or

mediastinal tumors. Hiatal hernias predispose patients to both intrinsic narrowing (strictures from GERD) and extrinsic compression (incarceration of a paraesophageal or sliding hernia). Disorders of **smooth muscle** (scleroderma, achalasia, Chagas' disease, diffuse esophageal spasm or "nutcracker" esophagus) and **striated muscle** (neuromuscular diseases, rabies, tetanus) cause motor dysphagia.

2. The symptom of dysphagia may be oropharyngeal or esophageal. **Oropharyngeal dysphagia** (throat and mouth etiologies) is suggested by a history of other oropharyngeal symptoms including nasal regurgitation, coughing on attempting to swallow and concomitant speech disturbances. Patients with recent stroke are particularly likely to have oropharyngeal dysphagia.

3. Esophageal dysphagia is caused by the other four etiological groups (blockage, intrinsic, extrinsic, and smooth/striated muscle). Blockage of the esophageal lumen, intrinsic narrowing, and extrinsic compression cause *mechanical* obstruction, while diseases of smooth and striated muscle cause *neuromuscular* dysphagia. Mechanical and neuromuscular types of dysphagia can usually be distinguished by a brief, but careful, history focusing on the type of food inducing dysphagia (solids, liquids), the pattern of dysphagia (intermittent, constant and/or progressive), and whether heartburn is present.

3. Dysphagia for solid foods only: This symptom suggests mechanical obstruction, as fluids are able to traverse the partially obstructed esophagus more easily than solids. If dysphagia for solid food is intermittent, it may be due to an esophageal (Schatzki) ring. With esophageal rings, the obstruction is mild, and only large food boluses are obstructed; hence the intermittent nature of symptoms. Progressive dysphagia with a history of heartburn suggests peptic esophagitis with or without a peptic stricture. Progressive dysphagia for solids without a history of heartburn is characteristic of esophageal tumors.

5. Dysphagia for both solids and liquids: This symptom is characteristic of neuromuscular dysphagia (motility disorder), or advanced mechanical obstruction preventing fluids from passing. Progressive motility-type dysphagia is usually due to achalasia. Pseudoachalasia, due to tumor infiltrating the myenteric plexus, is a rare cause of this symptom. Intermittent, episodic motility-type dysphagia with associated chest pain may indicate diffuse esophageal spasm. In patients from South America, chagasic achalasia should be considered. Progressive dysphagia with severe associated heartburn is seen with scleroderma.

6. Physical examination should include a search for cervical and supraclavicular lymph nodes and features of connective tissue disease. A barium esophagram typically is the first diagnostic test obtained. If a motility disorder is likely, esophageal manometry is obtained and, possibly, an upper GI endoscopy to rule out pseudoachalasia. If mechanical obstruction is seen on the barium study, an upper GI endoscopy with biopsy is indicated. Thoracic CT is useful for diagnosing the cause of extrinsic compression of the esophagus.

7. Here is a comprehensive list of the causes of dysphagia:

OH WHEN EATING BITES

Oropharyngeal dysphagia (stroke, Sjögren's, tongue
  paralysis/injury)
Herpes simplex/opportunistic infections (CMV,
  Candida)

Web
Hiatal hernia (incarcerated)
Esophageal spasm
Nutcracker esophagus

Extrinsic compression (thyroid mass, Zenker's
  diverticulum, aneurysm)
Achalasia
Trypanasomiasis (Chagas' disease)
Inflammatory bowel disease (Crohn's)
Neuromuscular diseases (myasthenia gravis,
  poliomyelitis, ALS, polymyositis)
GERD/peptic stricture

Burn (caustic ingestion)
Impacted foreign body
Tumor
Esophageal ring
Scleroderma

HEPATOMEGALY

BIG HEPATIC MASS

Budd-Chiari syndrome
Infections (viral hepatitis, EBV, Weil's disease, TB,
  amebic abscess, hydatid cyst)
Gaucher's disease/**G**lycogen storage diseases

Hepatic cysts (polycystic disease)
Extramedullary hematopoiesis (i.e., myeloproliferative diseases)
Primary biliary cirrhosis
Amyloidosis
Toxins
Iron overload (e.g., hemochromatosis)
Congestive heart failure

Malignancy (e.g., hepatoma, metastatic tumors, lymphoproliferative diseases, adenoma)
Alcohol
Sarcoidosis/granulomatous hepatitis
Schistosomiasis (vascular obstruction)

Notes

1. A palpable liver, hepatomegaly, may indicate acute infection, toxic damage, infiltration, metabolic disease, obstruction to bile drainage, or vascular congestion/obstruction. A palpable liver may also be detected in patients with COPD where there is downward displacement of the liver and, rarely, when there is an anatomic anomaly (Riedel's lobe).
2. The evaluation of hepatomegaly depends upon the rapidity of enlargement and presenting historical and clinical features. In general, assess liver enzymes, bilirubin, and hepatic synthetic function (prothrombin time, albumin), and follow up with imaging studies.

JAUNDICE

BILE

Biliary obstruction
Inherited disorders of bile metabolism
Liver parenchymal damage (infection, toxins)
Erythrocyte destruction

Notes

1. The pathophysiologic mechanisms of hyperbilirubinemia are outlined by the BILE mnemonic: (1) **biliary obstruction** (i.e., cholelithiasis), (2) **inherited disorders** of bile conjugation or excretion (i.e., Gilbert's, Dubin-Johnson, Crigler-Najjar and Rotor syndrome), (3) **liver parenchymal damage** (infection, toxins), and (4) **erythrocyte destruction** (hemolysis, ineffective erythropoiesis).

2. Jaundice results from hyperbilirubinemia and appears as yellowing of the skin and sclera. Other conditions may cause yellowing (carotenemia) or darkening (Addison's) of the skin, but do not cause scleral icterus. After obtaining a serum bilirubin level and confirming that skin pigmentation changes are due to jaundice, the next step is to fractionate the bilirubin into unconjugated ("indirect") and conjugated ("direct") fractions.

3. *Unconjugated* hyperbilirubinemia rarely causes bilirubin levels greater than 5 mg/dl; order hemolysis labs (haptoglobin, reticulocyte count, direct and indirect anti-globulin tests, etc.) if another cause is not apparent. Disorders that cause a predominantly unconjugated hyperbilirubinemia include erythrocyte abnormalities, sepsis (decreased hepatic uptake), CHF, and certain inherited conditions (Gilbert's, Crigler-Najjar types I and II).

4. If the patient has a predominantly *conjugated* hyperbilirubinemia, the next step is to differentiate between liver parenchymal damage and biliary obstruction. Liver parenchymal injury causes very high levels of transaminases: AST (SGOT) and ALT (SGPT). Biliary obstruction has a lesser increase in transaminases and a more remarkable elevation of alkaline phosphatase (and 5' nucleotidase, if obtained). If biliary obstruction is suspected, then differentiate between intra-hepatic and extra-hepatic biliary obstruction by imaging studies, often ultrasonography. Disorders that cause a predominantly conjugated hyperbilirubinemia include hepatocellular destruction (infection, drugs), biliary obstruction (stones, anomalies of the bile duct, cancer, sclerosing cholangitis), and a few inherited disorders of bile excretion (Dubin-Johnson, Rotor).

5. Here is a more complete list of etiologies of jaundice:

I'M PAGING MRS WHIPPLE STAT

Infection (e.g., viral hepatitis, sepsis, leptospirosis, *Clonorchis, Ascariasis*)
Medications/drugs

Postoperative cholestasis
Alpha-1 anti-trypsin deficiency
Gallstones

Injury/trauma (hemobilia)
Neoplasms (e.g., cholangiocarcinoma, periampullary carcinoma, carcinoma head of pancreas)
Granulomatous/infiltrative disease (e.g., sarcoidosis)

Malformation of the biliary tree (atresia, stricture, choledochal cyst, etc.)
Reye's syndrome
Sclerosing cholangitis

Wilson's disease
Hereditary diseases (Gilbert's, Dubin-Johnson, Rotor syndrome, Crigler-Najjar)
Iron overload
Pregnancy-related (cholestasis of pregnancy, pre-eclampsia, acute fatty liver of pregnancy)
Primary biliary cirrhosis
Laënnec's cirrhosis (alcoholic)
Erythrocyte destruction

Starvation/fasting
TPN
Autoimmune hepatitis
Toxins

Nausea and Vomiting

I VOMIT

Increased intracranial pressure/CNS disease

Vascular
Obstructive
Metabolic/toxic
Infectious
Traumatic

Notes

1. Nausea and vomiting are very common symptoms and may be associated with any of the causes of abdominal pain (see Abdominal Pain section). In fact, these symptoms often occur together. When nausea and vomiting are the primary symptoms, however, a different prioritization of diagnostic possibilities—summarized by the mnemonic I VOMIT (see also Pancreatitis section)—is appropriate. **Increased intracranial pressure**, as occurs with intracerebral hemorrhage, can cause nausea and vomiting. **Vascular** etiologies include mesenteric ischemia, myocardial ischemia, and migraine headache. **Obstruction** of the GI tract (e.g., adhesions, volvulus, intussusception) and pseudo-obstruction (e.g., scleroderma, gastroparesis) are common causes of nausea and vomiting. **Metabolic/toxic** causes include pregnancy, hypercalcemia, adrenal insufficiency, kidney failure, drugs, and diabetic ketoacidosis. **Infectious** etiologies include gastroenteritis, appendicitis, abscess, *Helicobacter pylori*, sepsis, and meningitis. Finally, **trauma** to the abdomen, either extrinsic or related to surgery, are easily recognized causes of nausea and vomiting.

2. Seek a history of headaches or neurological symptoms, as these may point toward a CNS cause of nausea and vomiting. Abdominal pain preceding the vomiting may help localize an intra-abdominal inflammatory process (e.g., epigastric pain with pancreatitis, right upper quadrant pain with cholecystitis, right lower quadrant pain with appendicitis). Undigested food in the vomitus may help localize the etiology to the stomach, but cannot distinguish mechanical obstruction from gastroparesis. Feculent vomitus suggests bowel obstruction or fistula.

3. In addition to performing a general physical examination, measure orthostatic changes in pulse and blood pressure to estimate the degree of dehydration. Orthostatic changes may also be due to autonomic dysfunction in diabetic patients, or due to drug therapy.

4. Abdominal examination should establish the presence or absence of distension. An absence of bowel sounds on auscultation may indicate an ileus or an inflammatory condition with peritonitis. Palpation of the abdomen helps distinguish the two, as localized tenderness with guarding is present in inflammatory conditions. The localization of pain and tenderness may indicate the organ system involved.

OH GOD AM I SICK

Obstetrical (pregnancy, hyperemesis gravida)
Hypercalcemia

Gastroenteritis (bacterial and viral)
Obstruction (adhesions, volvulus, intussusception, peptic strictures, tumors)
Diabetes (DKA, gastroparesis)

Adrenal insufficiency
Medications (opiates, antibiotics, NSAIDs, chemotherapeutic agents, antiarrhythmics)

Intra-abdominal inflammatory conditions (pancreatitis, cholecystitis, appendicitis, trauma)

Scleroderma (and other pseudo-obstructive states)
Ischemia (mesenteric, myocardial)
CNS disease (migraines, increased intracranial pressure, meningitis, stroke)
Kidney failure

Clinical Conditions or Diagnoses

PANCREATITIS

VOMIT

Vascular
Obstructive
Metabolic/toxic
Infectious
Traumatic

Notes

1. The VOMIT mnemonic (see Nausea and Vomiting section) can be used to classify the causes of pancreatitis. **Vascular** causes of pancreatitis include necrotizing

vasculitis, atheroemboli, and TTP. **Obstructive** causes of pancreatitis include biliary disease/cholelithiasis, pancreas divisum, ampullary malignancies. Crohn's disease, sphincter of Oddi dysfunction, Ascariasis infestation, duodenal diverticulum and (probably) cystic fibrosis. **Metabolic/toxic processes** causing pancreatitis include alcohol, drugs, renal failure, acute fatty liver, scorpion sting, Reye's syndrome, hypercalcemia, and hypertriglyceridemia. **Infectious** causes of pancreatitis include mumps, other viral infections, Reye's syndrome (also a toxic/metabolic process), Mycoplasma and Ascariasis (obstructs pancreatic outflow). **Traumatic** causes of pancreatitis include external trauma, ERCP, surgery, erosion of duodenal ulcer, and after renal transplantation (the latter also may be considered toxic/metabolic).

2. The most common causes of acute pancreatitis are (1) **biliary obstruction** by gall stones, (2) **alcohol** toxicity (these first two account for approximately 90% of cases), and (3) **drugs**, which account for about 5% of cases ("**BAD**"). Other iatrogenic causes (e.g., ERCP, post-operative, and calcium administration) are being increasingly recognized.

3. An important diagnostic test is the amylase level, although a normal level does not rule out pancreatitis. The lipase level may have somewhat greater sensitivity and specificity in the diagnosis of acute pancreatitis.

4. Other non-pancreatic conditions which cause an elevation of serum amylase include renal insufficiency, salivary gland disease, macroamylasemia, DKA, certain tumors (lung, esophagus, ovarian), burns, ectopic pregnancy, and other intra-abdominal disorders (perforated viscus, penetrating ulcer, peritonitis).

5. Serial measures of serum amylase are not helpful, and patients are best followed clinically. Urine amylase estimation is only helpful for making the diagnosis of macroamylasemia. In this condition, the amylase complex is too large to be filtered into the urine, and urine levels are low in contrast to elevated serum levels.

6. Ranson's criteria for pancreatitis may be used for prognosis. "**HELLO RANSON**" lists these factors:

On Admission	Within 48 Hours
Hyperglycemia (Glucose > 200 mg/dl)	**R**enal failure (BUN increase > 5 mg/dl)
Elevated AST > 250 u/l	**A**nemia (hematocrit drop > 10 mg/dl)
Leukocytosis (WBC > 16,000/mm^3)	**N**o calcium (< 8 mg/dl)
LDH > 350 u/l	**S**equestration (> 4 L fluid)
Older patients (Age > 55 years)	**O**xygen drop (PO$_2$ < 60 mmHg)
	No albumin (< 3.2 g/dl)

Patients with only one of these factors have an increased risk of complications; those with two risk factors may have a mortality rate as high as 20–30%; and those with six to seven risk factors have a nearly 100% mortality rate. In patients with gallstone-associated pancreatitis, the prognosis is generally better, and modified criteria have been proposed. Other indicators of poor prognosis include acidosis (base deficit > 4 mmol/L), hypotension (BP < 90 mmHg), tachycardia (heart rate > 130), oliguria (< 50 cc/hr) and hemorrhagic peritoneal fluid ("toxic broth"). An APACHE II score > 12 is also predictive of more severe disease, although it is a complex and seldom used calculation. The importance of risk stratification is that high-risk patients should be monitored more closely and are candidates for earlier interventional therapy (surgical, radiologic, endoscopic).

7. The treatment for pancreatitis is largely supportive, with fluid resuscitation and analgesia. The pancreas is rested by eliminating oral intake. Monitoring for complications (infection, hemorrhage, hemodynamic collapse, respiratory failure, hypocalcemia, hyperglycemia) is critical. There are no proven benefits for routine nasogastric suction, peritoneal lavage, administration of antibiotics, or therapy with other medications. In cases of gallstone pancreatitis, immediate removal of stones in severely ill patients may improve outcome. Other invasive therapies are reserved for severely ill patients with specific complications (e.g., abscess, pseudocyst, phlegmon).

8. The following mnemonic lists most of the causes and associations for pancreatitis:

BAD PANCREATITIS CRASHES HARD

Biliary disease (choledocholithiasis)
Alcohol
Drugs/toxins

Pancreas divisum
Ampullary malignancy (adenocarcinoma of the pancreas, primary ampullary, etc.)
Necrotizing vasculitis (lupus, polyarteritis nodosa)
Cystic fibrosis
Reye's syndrome
ERCP
Atheroemboli
Trauma
Infection (viral, parasites, bacterial)
TTP
Idiopathic/inherited
Surgery (postoperative pancreatitis, especially post cardiopulmonary bypass)

Crohn's disease
Renal failure
Acute fatty liver of pregnancy
Scorpion sting
Hypercalcemia
Erosion of duodenal ulcer
Sphincter of Oddi dysfunction

Hypertriglyceridemia
Ascariasis
Renal transplant
Duodenal diverticulum

X

RHEUMATOLOGY

Clinical Symptoms and Signs

ACUTE MONOARTHRITIS

HIS GOUT FIT*

Hemarthrosis (coagulopathy, e.g., hemophilia)
Infection (bacteria, [e.g., gonococcus], mycobacterial, fungal, Lyme disease, viral)
Systemic illness (Reiter's, SLE, rheumatoid arthritis, psoriasis, sarcoid, Behçet's)
Gout/pseudogout
Osteoarthritis
Ulcerative colitis/Crohn's
Trauma/foreign body synovitis

Fibrin deposition (palindromic arthritis)
Ischemic necrosis
Tumor (metastatic, primary)

---

* Differential diagnosis

Notes

1. Acute pain and swelling in a joint requires immediate evaluation and, in almost all cases, immediate arthrocentesis to rule out infection.

2. The age of the patient, history of other disease or symptoms (gastroenteritis), family history, and sexual history must be carefully evaluated. Physical examination is performed to look for signs of infection (skin changes) or evidence of other systemic illness. Consider culture of the throat, urethra, and rectum in individuals suspected of gonococcal infection.

3. Examine joint fluid by gram stain and polarized light initially, and send for a culture and cell count. Normal synovial fluid contains fewer than 110 cells/mm^3, most of which are mononuclear. Fluid is considered "noninflammatory" if it contains less than 3000 cells/mm^3. As the cell count increases, so does the suspicion of infection. Effusions with more than 100,000 WBC/mm^3 are considered septic, but there is a wide range of possible values. Careful examination of fluid for crystals may establish a diagnosis early and obviate the need for hospitalization. The presence of crystals, however, does *not* exclude infection, and if there is still a question of infection, the patient should be admitted for antibiotics until culture results are available. (See table in Inflammatory Polyarthritis section.)

4. A frequent diagnostic dilemma involves differentiating infections from other acute inflammatory arthritides. Patients should be admitted for intravenous antibiotics while awaiting culture results. NSAIDs should be withheld initially to judge the response to antibiotics alone.

INFLAMMATORY
POLYARTHRITIS

AGGRAVATED SYNOVIAL JTS*

Adult Stills' disease
Gout/pseudogout
Gonococcemia
Rheumatoid arthritis
Acute rheumatic fever
Vasculitis
Amyloidosis
Tuberculosis
Endocarditis
Dermatomyositis/polymyositis

Systemic lupus erythematosus
Yersinia, Campylobacter, Shigella (Reiter's)
Non-gonococcal urethritis (Reiter's)
Overlap syndromes (e.g., mixed connective tissue
   disease)
Viral infections (reactive)
Inflammatory bowel disease
AIDS
Lyme disease

Juvenile rheumatoid arthritis
Treponemal infection (syphilis)
Sarcoidosis

Also: scleroderma, polymyalgia rheumatica, psoriasis, intestinal bypass surgery, hemochromatosis

---

* This mnemonic provides the differential diagnosis.

Notes

1. A quick and easy etiologic way to look at inflammatory polyarthritis is as follows:
   a. Infection—direct infection of joint (bacteria, syphilis, TB, etc.)
   b. Crystal-induced (gout, pseudogout)
   c. Immunologic (RA, SLE, vasculitis, etc.)
   d. Reactive—in response to infection elsewhere in body (Reiter's syndrome, AIDS, etc.)
   e. Idiopathic (ankylosing spondylitis)
2. Work-up of inflammatory polyarthritis includes:
   a. Laboratory studies: CBC, ESR, CRP may help distinguish inflammatory from noninflammatory conditions.
   b. Synovial fluid aspiration is always indicated when either an infectious or crystal-induced inflammatory arthritis is being considered. Normal viscosity is such that when expressed from a syringe, each drop has a long tail or string attached. RBCs are not generally seen in synovial fluid except in a setting of hemarthrosis or trauma.

Synovial Fluid Characteristics

	Noninflammatory Arthritis	Crystal-Induced Arthritis	Infectious Arthritis
Appearance	Clear	Turbid, yellow	Turbid, opaque
WBC	< 3000 cells/ml	3000–50,000 cells/ml	> 50,000 cells/ml
Differential	Mostly mono-nuclear cells	Mostly PMNs	Mostly PMNs
Glucose	Normal (within 10–15 mg/dl of serum values)	Normal or low	Low
Protein	Normal	Normal or high	High
Viscosity	Good, stringing of fluid	Poor, no stringing	Poor, no stringing
Crystals	No	Yes	No
Gram stain/ culture	Negative	Negative	Positive

    c. Specific serologic tests: seek RF, ANA, complement levels, ASO titers, etc. only when a specific diagnosis is suggested; these tests are not useful as screening tools.

    d. Radiographic tests include:
- X-rays are indicated with history of trauma, suspected chronic infection, monoarticular involvement, or progressive disability. For inflammatory disorders, findings include primarily soft tissue swelling and periarticular demineralization. In chronic disease, joint space narrowing, calcification, osteophyte formation, and subchondral cysts may be seen.
- Radionuclide scans may show increased uptake in synovitis, infection, or malignancy. Osteonecrosis may be seen as decreased uptake.

CALCIUM PYROPHOSPHATE DIHYDRATE DEPOSITION DISEASE

HOW I GOT BAD CPPD

Hyperparathyroidism
Osteoarthritis
Wilson's disease

Iron overload

Gout
Ochronosis
Thyroid disease (hypothyroidism)

Bowel disease (Crohn's, ulcerative colitis)
Acromegaly
Diabetes

Congenital hypocalciuric hypercalcemia
Paget's disease
Post-traumatic
Disease resembling rheumatoid arthritis

Also: amyloidosis, hypophosphatemia, hereditary calcium pyrophosphate dihydrate deposition (CPPD)

Notes

1. There are numerous reported disease associations of CPPD (or pseudogout), but the importance of some is debatable, as rigorous, controlled studies are not

available. However, in patients with CPPD, consideration must be given to the possibility of an underlying disease process.

2. One characteristic feature of this disease is patellofemoral joint disease with a normal femoral/tibial joint.

3. Screening work-up usually includes TSH, calcium, and glucose levels. Also consider ferritin and ceruloplasmin.

CREST SYNDROME

CREST*

Calcinosis cutis
Raynaud's syndrome
Esophageal dysmotility
Sclerodactyly
Telangiectasia

---

* The mnemonic presents clinical characteristics.

Notes

1. Anti-centromere antibodies are seen in a high percentage of patients with CREST, but few patients with scleroderma/systemic sclerosis.

2. Calcinosis cutis describes irregular cutaneous papules that are firm and white.

3. Raynaud's phenomenon involves episodic vasoconstriction of the small arteries and arterioles of the digits. Triggers include cold, vibration, and stress. An initial vasoconstrictive event leads to *whitish* pallor in affected areas associated with the sensation of coldness, tingling, or pain. A cyanotic (*blue*) phase may occur, and the episode eventually resolves with a period of reactive hyperemia (*red*).

4. Esophageal dysmotility may manifest as dysphagia, heartburn, regurgitation, and/or a sensation of epigastric fullness.

5. Sclerodactyly involves taut, thinned skin over the digits, which may often have a tapered appearance. It eventually leads to diminished joint movement.

6. Telangiectasia features superficial cutaneous capillary malformations.

OSTEOARTHRITIS

I GOT MR. PAIN, DOC*

Idiopathic primary osteoarthritis

Gout
Occupational/sports
Trauma, acute/fracture

Metabolic (hemochromatosis, Wilson's, Gaucher's, ochronosis)
Rheumatoid arthritis

Psoriatic arthritis
Acromegaly/endocrine (hyperparathyroidism, DM, obesity, hypothyroid)
Infection
Neuropathic

Developmental (Legg-Calve-Perthes, congenital hip dislocation, etc.)
Osteopetrosis/osteochondritis
Calcium deposition disease

---

* Differential diagnosis

Notes

Osteoarthritis (OA) is a disease or pathology of movable, synovial joints. It is synonymous with degenerative joint disease
Heberden's nodes are bony enlargements of the distal interphalangeal joints. They are the most common form of idiopathic osteoarthritis.
Bouchard's nodes are bony enlargements of the proximal interphalangeal joints.

1. OA may be classified as primary or secondary. *Primary* OA occurs in the absence of an identifiable underlying etiology. *Secondary* OA is due to an underlying condition or disease.

2. Locations of OA:

   a. Interphalangeal joints: Heberden's and Bouchard's nodes

   b. Hip: most cases are secondary and due to congenital or developmental defects.

   c. Knee:

- **Varus** deformity (bow-legged) due to medial compartment OA
- **Valgus** deformity (knock-kneed) due to lateral compartment OA
- **Chondromalacia**, a syndrome of knee pain, usually occurs in younger patients and is not generally progressive to true OA.

   d. Spine:

- **Spondylosis**—degenerative *disk* disease
- **Diffuse idiopathic skeletal hyperostosis**—calcification and ossification of paraspinous ligaments
- **Osteoarthritis of the spine**—degeneration of movable, synovial-lined spinal joints

3. Clinical signs and symptoms

   a. Pain has gradual onset, dull aching. Joint tenderness and pain occur with range of motion.

   b. Morning stiffness is not prominent, as in inflammatory rheumatic disease.

   c. Crepitus is a grinding sound or sensation heard or felt as joint is moved.

   d. Joint enlargement may be due to soft tissue swelling/effusion or osteophytes.

   e. Joint deformity, such as Heberden's and Bouchard's nodes, varus or valgus angulation

4. Work-up of OA

   a. X-rays of affected joints—may be normal, or show joint space narrowing, subchrondral sclerosis, subchondral cysts, and marginal osteophytes.

   b. Routine laboratory tests help identify causes of secondary OA, including ESR, CBC, serum chemistries, urinalysis.

   c. Synovial fluid: mild leukocytosis (< 2000 WBC/ml, < 25% PMNs), no crystals, good mucin clot.

5. **Charcot joints**—secondary OA due to underlying neurologic disease.

RHEUMATOID ARTHRITIS

RF RISES

Rheumatoid factor elevated
Finger/hand joints involved

Rheumatoid nodules
Involvement of three or more joints
Stiffness, morning
Erosions/decalcifications on X-rays
Symmetric (bilateral) arthritis

Notes

Rheumatoid arthritis (RA) is a chronic multi-system disorder characterized by inflammatory joint disease, usually symmetric.

1. Diagnostic criteria
   a. Four of the seven criteria above are needed to diagnose RA.
   b. Patients with two or more other clinical diagnoses are *not* excluded.
2. Elevation of serum **rheumatoid factor** can be determined by any method that has < 5% false positive rate.
3. **Finger/hand joint involvement** includes arthritic changes in the wrist and the metacarpophalangeal (MCP) or proximal interphalangeal (PIP) joints.
4. **Rheumatoid nodules** are firm, round, subcutaneous nodules over the joints, extensor surfaces, or bony prominences. They are seen in 20–25% of patients.
5. Multiple joint involvement (of three or more) refers to soft tissue swelling or joint effusions, not just osteophytes. Fourteen possible areas are described: right or left proximal interphalangeal, metacarpophalangeal, wrist, elbow, knee, ankle, and metatarsophalangeal joints.
6. **Morning stiffness** is defined as a joint stiffness upon awakening that persists 1 hour before maximal improvement.
7. Radiographic findings in hand and wrist x-rays must include **erosions** or bony decalcification in or adjacent to affected joints.
8. **Symmetry** means simultaneous involvement of the same joint bilaterally.
9. Signs and symptoms:
   a. Joint manifestations
      * Generalized: pain, joint swelling, effusion, warmth, and limited range of motion.
      * Cervical spine: most serious is atlantoaxial subluxation. May cause nerve root impingement, spinal cord symptoms, or even lower brainstem problems.
      * Cricoarytenoid joint: impairs vocal cord mobility, cause hoarseness.
      * Shoulder: synovitis and rotator cuff injury.
      * Elbow: rheumatoid nodules on extensor surface of forearm lead to olecranon bursitis.
      * Hand/wrist: typically distal interphalangeal (DIP) joints are spared. **Swan neck deformity** is flexion at the DIP and MCP joints and hyperextension at the PIP joints. **Boutonniere deformity** is DIP hyperextension

with PIP flexion. **Carpal tunnel syndrome** is not uncommon. **Ulnar drift** is a deformity characterized by PIP flexion and deviation of the fingertips toward the ulna.

- Hip: may manifest with groin pain. Severe involvement is rare (5%).
- Knee: very common. **Baker's cyst** is a posterior herniation of synovium and fluid from the knee into the popliteal fossa.
  - Ankle/foot: Common in both ankle and foot. **Cock-up toe** deformity occurs at the metatarsophalangeal joint.

b. Systemic manifestations include weight loss, fatigue, achiness, anorexia, malaise.

c. Other organ involvement

i. Rheumatoid nodules: see number 4, previous page

ii. Eye manifestations: **Sicca complex** is burning, gritty eye sensation; dry mouth; and salivary gland enlargement. Episcleritis and scleritis may also occur.

iii. Cardiac: rarely clinically significant, but include pericarditis and inflammatory granulomas.

iv. Pulmonary: pleuritis, pleural effusions, interstitial fibrosis and nodules. **Caplan's syndrome** consists of interstitial fibrosis and multiple nodules.

v. Neurologic: entrapment neuropathies (carpal tunnel), occasional vasculitic complications.

vi. Hematologic: anemia, thrombocytosis (500–700 K), mild leukocytosis. **Felty's syndrome** is a combination of RA, thrombocytopenia, leukopenia, and splenomegaly.

vii. Vasculitis: cutaneous, neuropathic, or visceral involvement with ischemic complications.

10. Diagnostic work-up

a. CBC—normochromic, normocytic anemia. Also thrombocytosis, elevated ESR, increased IgG, and even eosinophilia.

b. Rheumatoid factor—positive in 70–80%. Nonspecific. ANA positive (25% of patients) and VDRL false positive (5–10%).

c. Synovial fluid—WBC 5000–25,000, mostly PMNs. Glucose low and complement levels low. No crystals.

d. X-rays—approximate symmetric involvement, osteopenia/decalcification, soft tissue swelling, bony erosions, joint space narrowing.

Systemic Sclerosis (Scleroderma)

SCLERODERMA*

Skin changes
Cardiac involvement
Lung involvement
Esophageal dysfunction
Raynaud's phenomenon
Obstruction, pseudo-
Dry eyes/mouth
Endocrine (hypothyroidism)
Renal failure
Myopathy/myositis
Arthritis

---

* Clinical characteristics

Notes

1. **Skin changes** include early swelling, particularly of the fingers and hands. Later, skin becomes firm and thickened. Chronically, skin becomes thin and atrophic. Skin over the fingers become taut, and contractures limit movement. Other cutaneous manifestations include telangiectasia, subcutaneous calcifications, salt-and-pepper pigmentary changes, abnormal nail bed capillaries, and skin ulcers.

2. **Cardiac involvement** includes pericarditis, pericardial effusion, heart failure, and heart block/arrhythmia. Myocardial fibrosis causing cardiomyopathy occurs in < 10%.

3. **Lung involvement** occurs in two-thirds of patients and is often manifested by exertional dyspnea and dry, nonproductive cough. Additional complications include pulmonary fibrosis, aspiration pneumonia, decreased vital capacity, and decreased lung compliance. Pulmonary hypertension in the absence of fibrosis can occur in < 10%.

4. **Gastrointestinal dysmotility** is related to neuromuscular dysfunction. This may manifest as heartburn, dysphagia, reflux/regurgitation, delayed gastric

emptying, bloating, abdominal pain, and pseudo-obstruction. Bacterial over-growth can lead to malabsorption syndrome.

5. Hypothyroidism may occur and is due to either antithyroid antibodies or fibrosis.

6. Renal failure may occur insidiously or as a renal crisis. Renal crisis is char-acterized by malignant hypertension, hypertensive encephalopathy, severe headache, retinopathy, seizures and left ventricular failure. This occurs due to overactivation of the renin-angiotensin system. Renal failure is the leading cause of death in systemic sclerosis.

7. Muscular effects of scleroderma include disuse atrophy, myopathy without enzyme abnormalities, and, rarely, a polymyositis-like syndrome.

8. Polyarthritis is manifested by pain, swelling, and stiffness—particularly in the hands, fingers, and knees in more than 50% of patients. Tendon sheath fibrosis may become a problem, and can lead to carpal tunnel syndrome when it occurs in the wrist.

SYSTEMIC LUPUS ERYTHEMATOSUS

ORDER HIS ANA

Oral ulcers
Rash (malar)
Discoid rash
Exaggerated photosensitivity
Renal disease

Hematologic abnormalities
Immunologic abnormalities
Serositis

Arthralgias/arthritis (nonerosive)
Neurologic disease
Anti-nuclear antibody

Notes

1. The diagnosis of SLE depends upon the presence of four or more of the above 11 criteria. The disease, however, may involve any organ system.
2. The findings of oral ulcers, malar rash, discoid rash, exaggerated photosensitivity, and arthritis are obtained by history and physical examination. Neurologic criteria include seizures and psychosis (in the absence of other drugs or precipitants). Renal disease is defined as persistent proteinuria or cellular casts. Serositis may be manifested as pleuritis or pericarditis. Immunologic criteria for diagnosis include a positive LE cell preparation, anti-DNA antibodies, anti-SM antibodies, or a false-positive serologic test for syphilis. Hematologic criteria include hemolytic anemia, leukopenia, lymphopenia, or thrombocytopenia.
3. Other manifestations of SLE include fever, pancreatitis, hepatitis, retinal disease, myocardial disease (myocarditis, endocarditis), gastrointestinal disease, pulmonary disease (diffuse infiltrates, vasculitis), and coagulopathy (lupus anticoagulant).

VASCULITIS

WHAM! ANGIITIS*

Wegener's granulomatosis
Hypersensitivity vasculitis (Henoch-Schönlein)
Associated with systemic disease, rheumatic disease, neoplasm
Mucocutaneous lymph node syndrome (Kawasaki's)

Allergic angiitis (Churg-Strauss disease)
Nodosa, polyarteris
Giant cell arteritis (temporal arteritis)
Iatrogenic/drug-induced
Infection
Takayasu's arteritis
Isolated CNS vasculitis
Serum sickness

---

* Differential diagnosis

Notes

Vasculitis is a disorder characterized by inflammation and damage to blood vessels, often resulting in ischemia to tissues supplied by affected vessels. It may occur as a primary manifestation of disease or in combination with other pathologic processes, and may be limited to one organ or affect multiple organs.

1. **Wegener's granulomatosis** vasculitis usually affects *small* vessels and is classically associated with upper and lower respiratory tract involvement and glomerulonephritis (see Wegener's section).
2. **Hypersensitivity vasculitis** is a broad group of disorders believed to be due to a reaction to a particular (endogenous or exogenous) antigen and involving *small* vessels.
   a. Henoch-Schönlein purpura—palpable purpura (usually on buttocks and lower extremities), arthralgias, GI symptoms, and glomerulonephritis. More common in children.
   b. **Associated with other primary diseases**—often connective tissue diseases (SLE, RA, Sjögren's syndrome), malignancies (lymphoid or reticuloendothelial, hairy cell leukemia), or other illnesses (cryoglobulinemia, primary biliary cirrhosis, alpha$_1$ antitrypsin deficiency, ulcerative colitis, and intestinal bypass surgery).
   c. **Iatrogenic/drug-induced**—penicillin and sulfa may induce a serum sickness-like reaction.
   d. **Infection**—subacute bacterial endocarditis, Epstein-Barr virus, hepatitis
   e. **Serum sickness**—fever, urticaria, arthralgias, and lymphadenopathy 7–10 days after primary exposure or 2–4 days after secondary exposure to foreign protein.
3. **Mucocutaneous lymph node syndrome** (Kawasaki's)—acute; fever, cervical adenitis, conjunctival edema, orolingual and palmar erythemia, fingertip desquamation; occurs in children. Danger is later development of coronary artery aneurysms. Treat with IV immunoglobulin and aspirin.
4. **Allergic angiitis** (Churg-Strauss) is characterized by hypereosinophilia, allergic rhinitis/asthma, and *small-medium* vessel vasculitis involving two or more extrapulmonary sites.
5. **Polyarteritis nodosa** (PAN)—*small-medium* vessel arteritis involving multiple organ systems, including renal (60%), musculoskeletal (64%), peripheral nervous system (51%), GI tract (44%), skin (43%), cardiac (36%), genitourinary (25%), and CNS (23%).
6. **Giant cell arteritis** (temporal arteritis)—*large* vessel arteritis associated with fever, anemia, headache, and elevated ESR. Usually in elderly patient. Danger is development of amaurosis fugax and retinal ischemia. Diagnosed clinically and confirmed by temporal artery biopsy. Treated with prednisone.
7. **Takayasu's arteritis**—*medium-large* vessel arteritis, more prevalent in East Asia, and more likely in the aortic arch or its direct branches. Manifestations are usually ischemia in distribution of affected arteries (including cerebral infarction).

8. **Isolated CNS vasculitis**—usually *arteriolitis*, but any size vessel may be affected. Diagnosed by angiography and brain/meningeal biopsy. Associated with CMV, syphilis, bacteria, varicella-zoster virus, Hodgkin's disease, and amphetamine abuse.

WEGENER'S GRANULOMATOSIS

LUNG HEAD*

Lung/pulmonary vasculitis
Upper respiratory tract disease, sinusitis
Neuropathy, cranial or peripheral
Glomerulonephritis/renal disease

Heart involvement
Eye involvement
Arthralgias/arthritis
Dermatologic lesions

---

* Clinical characteristics

Notes

1. Classic clinical presentation:
    a. Upper respiratory tract involvement—sinusitis, nasal drainage
    b. Lower respiratory tract/pulmonary involvement—cough, hemoptysis, dyspnea
    c. Renal involvement—glomerulonephritis, proteinuria, hematuria
2. Neurologic signs/symptoms occur in 22% of patients. Granulomatous involvement of cranial nerves or mononeuritis multiplex due to vasculitis may occur. Less likely is CNS vasculitis or cerebral granuloma.
3. Cardiac manifestations (12% of patients) include pericarditis, coronary vasculitis, or, rarely, cardiomyopathy.

4. Ophthalmologic involvement is fairly common (60%): conjunctivitis, episcleritis, scleritis, uveitis, vasculitis, and/or retro-orbital mass resulting in proptosis.

5. Joint-related symptoms include arthralgias/joint pain (up to 50%). True synovitis is rare.

6. Cutaneous manifestations of Wegener's are seen in 45% of cases and include papules, vesicles, purpura, ulcers, or subcutaneous nodules.

7. An important diagnostic distinction is that between Wegener's and lymphomatous granulomatosis. While the former is a multisystem inflammatory vasculitis, the latter is a diffuse infiltration of atypical lymphocytoid cells which is seen in the lung, skin, CNS, and kidney. Lymphomatosis evolves into malignant lymphoma in 50% of cases, while Wegener's does not.

XI

NEUROLOGY

The key to a good differential diagnosis is to start with a broad, all-inclusive differential based on the major points of the case and narrow it down logically to a smaller, "working" differential based on the specifics of the case. If the patient's signs/symptoms become atypical, or new information becomes available, you can go back to the broad differential; in this way, you will not miss unusual presentations of disease. Consider a 50-year-old man with hypertension, diabetes, and hyperlipidemia presenting with stroke: the expanded differential should include all causes of stroke, but the working differential features atherothrombotic disease, hemorrhage, and embolism as likely etiologies. If the CT scan shows a mass lesion, then you'd better return to the broad differential to include tumor and brain abscess. If the patient develops a fever and is found to have a sedimentation rate of 100, then you should return to the expanded differential and retrieve vasculitis and infection to add to your working differential.

Without a complete initial differential diagnosis, or a return to the initial differential when a typical case becomes atypical, you will miss diagnoses.

General Considerations

How to Make a Broad Differential Diagnosis

Despite the stereotype of neurology as a mysterious and arcane "black box," there are several effective methods to help any physician make a complete differential diagnosis for neurological disease.

Differential by Etiology

The MEDICINE DOC mnemonic is a useful starting place to develop a complete neurologic differential diagnosis. To review:

Metabolic disease (e.g., metabolic encephalopathy, leukodystrophy, Wilson's disease)

Endocrine disease (e.g., diabetic neuropathy, myxedema coma, hypoglycemic seizures)

Drugs/medicines (e.g., iatrogenic, accidental, self-administered)

Infections (e.g., meningitis, herpes encephalitis, HIV dementia, neurosyphilis)

Congenital abnormalities (e.g., spina bifida, Chiari malformations, muscular dystrophy)

Immunologic disease (e.g., vasculitis, myasthenia gravis)

Neoplasms (e.g., primary tumors, metastatic disease)

Exotic ("strange" diseases of uncertain etiology, e.g., multiple sclerosis, Guillain-Barré)

Degenerative processes (e.g., Alzheimer's, Parkinson's)

Occupational exposures (e.g., environmental or occupational toxins, trauma)

Cardiovascular (e.g., infarction, hemorrhage, embolism, aneurysm, arteriovenous malformation)

Differential by Anatomy

A detailed understanding of neuroanatomy, although useful in precisely localizing lesions, pinpointing diagnoses, and impressing/boring colleagues during rounds, is not required to make basic differentials. The simplest method is to start at the muscle and work back anatomically to the cerebral cortex. Examples of an anatomic differential for "weakness" are in parentheses:

1. Muscle (polymyositis)
2. Neuromuscular junction (myasthenia gravis)
3. Peripheral nerve (Guillain-Barré)
4. Nerve plexus (brachial amyotrophy)
5. Nerve root (disc herniation)
6. Meninges/subarachnoid space (arachnoiditis)
7. Spinal cord (spinal cord tumor)
8. Brainstem (pontine infarction)
9. Subcortical structures—basal ganglia, thalamus (lacunar infarction—internal capsule)
10. Cortical structures—cerebrum, cerebellum (middle cerebral artery infarction)

How to Make a "Working" Differential Diagnosis

Essential in the development of a useful working differential diagnosis is taking clinical characteristics from the case in point and using them to narrow down the broad differential. Herein lies the art of diagnosis: how do you know when a history of alcohol abuse is helpful in making the diagnosis of alcohol withdrawal seizure, or simply a "red herring" distracting you from the correct diagnosis of meningitis? If things don't fit, *go back to the broad differential.* Make sure nothing has been overlooked.

Differential by Time Course

In many diseases, and particularly in neurologic diseases, the time course of symptomatology is critical to intelligently narrowing down the differential. Different etiologies are suggested by different time courses. Intermittent symptoms with complete resolution between episodes invoke a different set of diagnoses than chronic, gradually progressive symptoms. A history of headache with nausea and vomiting might be due to migraine in a patient with the first time course, but the second course is more consistent with a brain tumor. It also is possible for a history of episodic symptoms to be gradually progressive (such as crescendo transient ischemic attacks). Take a careful history of the timing of the symptoms.

A good history of the time course includes not only whether the symptoms are intermittent or continuous, but also the following information: whether the symptoms were maximal at onset, rapidly progressive, or progressing in a stepwise fashion; what factors exacerbate/precipitate symptoms and what factors ameliorate symptoms; if episodic, the duration and frequency of the episodes; and if and in what order associated symptoms occur.

Here is a general overview of the relationship between time course and the onset of initial symptoms and etiology.

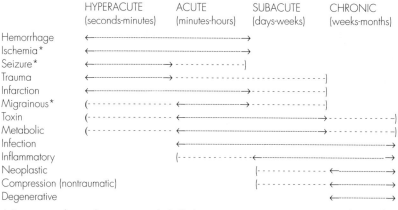

* Denotes etiologies that are particularly likely to cause intermittent symptoms with complete resolution of symptoms between episodes

Differential by Age of Patient

It is helpful and important to narrow the differential diagnosis based on the age of the patient. An acute neurologic deficit has an entirely different list of likely etiologies in a 90-year-old than it does in a 20-year-old. In general, congenital, traumatic, migrainous, and infectious etiologies are more frequent in younger patients. Older patients are more likely to have symptoms related to ischemic, neoplastic, chronic compression, or degenerative diseases.

Differential by Neuroanatomic Localization

The most basic distinction in neuroanatomy is whether a lesion is located in the central nervous system (the brain and spinal cord) or the peripheral nervous system (peripheral nerves, nerve roots, neuromuscular junction and muscle). Some clinical examination findings are useful in making this distinction. In the example below diagnoses suggested by a given combination of exam findings and neurologic localization are in parentheses.

Factors Distinguishing Location of Injury

Exam Finding	CNS (brain/spinal cord)	PNS (nerves/roots/NMJ/muscle)
• *Cranial Nerve Exam*		
Visual loss	Field cut (occipital infarct)	Monocular loss (retinal artery occlusion)
Optic disc	Normal or bilateral abnormality (increased intracranial pressure)	May be abnormal on one side only (optic neuritis)
Facial weakness	Forehead spared (frontal infarct)	Forehead weak (Bell's palsy)
• *Motor Exam*		
Muscle tone	Acutely decreased, later increased	Decreased
Atrophy	Absent	Acutely absent, later present
Fasciculations	Absent	Acutely absent, later present
Deep tendon reflexes	Acutely hypoactive, later hyperactive	Hypoactive
Babinski	May be present	Absent
Clonus	May be present	Absent
	(multiple sclerosis, cerebral infarct, intracranial bleed, brain tumor, spinal cord injury)	(radiculopathy, neuropathy, myopathy, myasthenia)
Both upper and lower motor neuron signs	(amytrophic lateral sclerosis [ALS], cervical stenosis)	

Differential by Risk Factors and Coexisting Medical Conditions

Making a differential diagnosis solely on the basis of risk factors is foolhardy, to say the least. However, risk factors such as environmental exposures, medications, drugs/alcohol, and coexisting medical conditions are helpful in narrowing down to a good working differential. For example, diabetes, ~~tension~~, atrial fibrillation, and smoking are all risk factors associated with ~~ce~~bral infarction. Pre-existing cancer might suggest several risk factors, including metastatic disease, immunosuppression, and exposure to chemotherapeutic drugs and/or radiation, each of which will mold the differential in a slightly different way. Immunosuppressed status by itself suggests a whole host of infections which would not normally be considered in an immunocompetent patient. Intravenous drug abuse increases the possibility of bacterial endocarditis, spinal epidural abscess, and brain abscess, as well as HIV. Uremia can lead to encephalopathy, seizures, myoclonus, and neuropathy. Organ transplantation has a whole host of disorders associated with dysfunction of the transplanted organ, immunosuppression, and side effects of multiple medications.

Use these factors as hints and suggestions, but do not rely on them to make the diagnosis. For example, the alcoholic who just seized and now has a hemiparesis may have had an alcohol withdrawal seizure with a post-ictal Todd's paralysis, but don't miss the subdural hematoma he got falling down the stairs, which is the real reason he seized and is hemiparetic. If you jump to the conclusion that he has had "just" an alcohol withdrawal seizure, then you may find yourself unhappily awakened to see him herniating in the middle of the night.

How to Do a Good Neurologic Examination

There are several aspects of the neurological work-up that are unique and must be considered when evaluating a patient with neurological disease. **The history is critical.** The history is where you will get information regarding the exact symptoms the patient experiences or experienced and the time course of these symptoms. In many cases, the history makes the diagnosis, and the examination serves merely as a confirmation of your historical diagnosis.

Realize, however, that the symptoms the patient reports can sometimes (often?) be vague and difficult to interpret. It is in these cases that the examination plays a key role. A patient may complain of visual loss in the left eye, but on examination, it becomes clear that the patient actually has a left homonymous hemianopia. This distinction is of great value, for monocular visual loss indicates disease in the eye or the blood supply to the retina (from the carotid artery), while a left visual field cut suggests pathology in the right occipital lobe or its blood supply (from the vertebral-basilar arteries). The work-up and treatment thus are significantly altered by the exam findings, which help to clarify the patient's interpretation of his/her neurologic deficit.

If something is found on exam that is inconsistent with the patient's history, this does not necessarily imply malingering, but rather a difficulty in accurately describing symptoms. Always be sure you understand what the patient is trying to describe. Some patients complain of weakness, when they really mean numbness, and vice versa. A patient may complain of an acute or subacute onset of

...xamination shows severe atrophy. Atrophy is a sign of lower ...ease, but it is not present acutely. In this case, further question-...ecessary to try to elicit a more chronic (and perhaps subtle) his-...ss (another possibility is a pre-existing chronic weakness with a ...new, acute insult).

From ...e examples you can see that the neurologic history and examination are interrelated and that, while the history often suggests the diagnosis, it is important to synthesize the information from both to come up with the correct answer. In addition, realize that if a basic neurologic function is impaired, it is not easy to reliably test higher neurologic functions; i.e., if a patient's arm is paralyzed or paretic, then fine motor coordination is difficult to assess; likewise, it would be unfair to label a patient as having severely impaired memory if the patient is aphasic.

The Mental Status Examination

A good mental status examination leaves no doubt about the patient's **level of arousal** for the next examiner. Terms like "sleepy," "lethargic," "stuporous" may mean slightly different things to different examiners. The best mental status exam simply states what the patient can or cannot do. For example, "The patient was awake, watching television, and speaking normally," or "The patient was asleep, arousable to tactile stimulation, but would fall back to sleep if unstimulated."

Remember to check basic and objective information. Is the patient **oriented to person, place, and time?** Assess the patient's **attention**. This is most easily done by having the patient repeat a series of random numbers, starting with three numbers in 3 seconds and working up until the patient is no longer able to correctly repeat them (normal is five to seven numbers in as many seconds). This is known as the *digit span*. If a patient's attention is impaired, as demonstrated by a digit span of less than 5, then more complicated mental status testing may be difficult to interpret. For instance, a patient with a digit span of 3 is not likely to be able to remember three objects in 5 minutes, but this does not necessarily imply a primary memory problem and may just represent poor attention to the examiner. Impaired attention may mean simply that the patient is preoccupied or anxious or may signify an acute confusional state or encephalopathy.

Speech is important to assess for both fluency (language output) and comprehension (language input). An impairment of smooth and fluent output suggests dysfunction of the dominant (usually left) frontal lobe (Broca's area), while fluent output with an inability to understand spoken language indicates damage to the dominant parietal-temporal area (Wernicke's area). Difficulty with both fluency and comprehension is usually the result of a more extensive dominant hemisphere lesion (such as a middle cerebral artery infarct).

Cranial Nerve Examination

Objective assessment of many of the cranial nerves (CNs) is possible, and thus brainstem function may be assessed even in comatose or otherwise uncooperative patients. Abnormalities in the cranial nerve exam usually suggest underlying brainstem pathology.

CN I: Sense of smell usually is not tested, but may be by asking the patient to identify a characteristic aroma with eyes closed (e.g., coffee, flowers).

CN II: Check *visual fields* to confrontation (Can patient see movement in all fields? Can patient count fingers in all fields?) and look for consensual *pupillary reactivity.*

CN III, IV, VI: Have the patient follow the movement of light in all directions.

Doll's eye maneuver (oculocephalic)—This is most useful in patients whose consciousness is impaired. A normal or positive response occurs when vigorously rotating the patient's head to one side, and the eyes deviate to the opposite side. An abnormal or negative response is when the eyes do not move in the orbits regardless of head position—the doll's eyes are absent. A fully conscious patient may be able to voluntarily override this reflex, resulting in a "false" negative result.

Cold calorics (oculovestibular)—ear canals are inspected for a clear view of the eardrums, the patient's head is hyperextended about 30°, and ice-cold water is irrigated into one ear canal. A normal or positive response in an awake patient is deviation of the eyes toward the irrigated ear and nystagmus beating away from the irrigated ear. (Since awake patients can voluntarily move their eyes, and since cold calorics can be quite nauseating, calorics are seldom indicated in awake patients.) A normal or positive response in a comatose patient is deviation of the eyes toward the irrigated ear, with no nystagmus. An abnormal or negative response shows no eye deviation. After 5 minutes, repeat the test with the opposite ear.

CN V: Ask the patient to close his/her eyes, touch (or use a pin to prick) the patient's face on the forehead, cheek, and chin on either side, and have the patient identify specifically or point to the place touched.

CN VII: Ask the patient to close his/her eyes tightly and look for the ability to "bury the eyelashes" symmetrically. Look for a symmetric smile. Ask the patient to "puff out his/her cheeks" and try to gently push the air out of the cheeks with your fingers. Ask the patient to clench his/her teeth together and look for symmetric contraction of the platysma muscle (stretches from the chin/jaw to the clavicles).

CN V/VII: *Corneal test*—A light wisp of cotton or tissue is brushed gently against the cornea, approaching from the side (not from the front). A positive response is eye closure/blinking. This should be done on one eye, then the other. Corneals may be absent in patients with a history of contact lens use. This test is not routinely performed in awake patients.

CN VIII: Whisper numbers (or letters) into the patient's ear from a distance of about 1 foot and note if the patient can repeat the numbers.

CN IX/X: *Gag test*—Using a Q-tip or tongue depressor, touch the back of the oropharynx on one side, then the other, and look for a gag with symmetric palate elevation. If the patient is intubated, a Q-tip can still be used. Pulling on the endotracheal tube is not recommended as a method for testing the gag reflex. A decreased or absent gag sometimes can be found in otherwise normal patients, but an asymmetric gag usually is indicative of brainstem pathology.

CN XI: Against resistance, have the patient shrug his/her shoulders up (trapezius) and turn his/her head to one side (sternocleidomastoid). Remember, difficulty turning the head to the right indicates a weak left sternocleidomastoid, and vice versa.

CN XII: Ask the patient to stick out his/her tongue. The tongue will deviate toward the weak side.

Motor Examination

Although the motor examination as typically discussed relies significantly on patient cooperation, there is a lot of objective information that can be elicited by a skilled examiner.

Muscle bulk is very objective, and focal *atrophy* or *fasciculations* are a sign of chronic lower motor neuron disease (ALS, neuropathy, radiculopathy, sometimes myopathy).

Muscle tone can be assessed by passively moving a joint through its full range of motion. *Flaccid tone* offers little or no resistance, and the movement will seem limp. This demonstrates either an acute upper motor neuron lesion or a lower motor neuron lesion. *Spastic tone* offers more resistance the faster the movement. Spasticity is seen with subacute or chronic upper motor neuron injury (spinal cord injury, cerebral infarct, brain tumor, multiple sclerosis, ALS). *Rigidity* shows equal resistance throughout the entire range, regardless of the velocity of the movement. Occasionally rigidity has a ratchety quality, which is referred to as *cogwheeling* (Parkinsonism, other basal ganglia disease). Experience aids greatly in the accurate evaluation of muscle tone.

Pronator drift is an excellent method of testing for subtle corticospinal weakness. The patient is asked to hold both arms fully extended in front of him/herself with the palms up. The palms should be level and not touching each other. The patient must then maintain this position with the eyes closed. A positive drift (and hence, evidence of corticospinal weakness) is characterized by not only a downward movement of the affected side, but also pronation of that extremity.

Subtle lower extremity weakness is suggested by **external rotation of the hip** at rest.

Direct **strength testing** of individual muscles is graded on the following scale:

0	No movement
1	Twitch or faint movement
2	Movement but not against gravity
3	Full movement against gravity but not against resistance
4	Movement against partial resistance
5	Movement against full resistance

A "+" or "−" sign often is used to denote smaller variations of strength (e.g., slight weakness against full resistance would be 5−. *Paralysis* or *plegia* means that there is no observable movement. *Paresis* means there is weakness but still observable movement.

Another part of the motor exam that assesses strength without direct one-on-one muscle testing is **functional testing**. Can the patient easily rise from a sitting position to a standing position without pushing up with the arms? An inability to do this suggests proximal lower extremity weakness. Can the patient walk up steps? Stand on one leg? Hop on one leg? Being able to stand on one's tip toes implies at least 4 to 4+ power in the gastrocnemius. Being able to stand on one's heels suggests at least the same degree of power in the anterior tibialis.

Does the patient have a **resting tremor** (Parkinsonism)? Does the patient have a tremor when forced to maintain posture, such as when the hands are outstretched? This is called a **postural tremor** and is often physiologic, but may be familial (essential tremor).

Cerebellar Examination

Can the patient rapidly and alternately pat the palm of the hand and the dorsum of the hand on a surface? This is the **rapid alternating movement test**, which assesses the cerebellum's ability to coordinate agonists and antagonists. Impairment of this is termed dysdiadochokinesis.

An **intention tremor** is a tremor that worsens with motion toward a particular point. It is checked for by having the patient rapidly alternate pointing (and touching) the examiner's outstretched finger and the patient's nose (**finger-nose-finger test**).

The **heel-knee-shin test** involves touching one heel to the opposite knee and smoothly moving the heel down the opposite shin to the ankle and back up to the knee. Normally this is a steady movement, but patients with ataxia wobble the moving leg from side to side.

An inability to perform any of these tests (in the absence of significant motor weakness) suggests ipsilateral cerebellar dysfunction.

Gait and Stance Examination

Gait and stance may be observed casually when the patient is walking to the examining area. Normal gait has a narrow stance, fluid movement, and symmetric arm swinging. Normal stance is steady with feet side by side and no swaying. Specific maneuvers can be tested later in the exam.

Tandem gait is tested by having the patient walk heel to toe in a straight line, and a difficulty with this (ataxic gait) suggests midline cerebellar dysfunction. Obese and elderly patients may have some difficulty with tandem gait without specific cerebellar disease.

Ataxic gait is characterized by unsteadiness, swaying, walking with the feet widely apart, and an inability to perform tandem gait.

Hemiparetic gait demonstrates decreased movement of the weak side, with the patient having to lean away from the paretic leg and swing it back to front (circumduction). The arm swing usually is decreased on the affected side, and the arm may be held in a flexed posture.

Parkinsonian gait classically has a stooped forward posture with small shuffling steps and a tendency to fall over backward (retropulsion). Turns are not made with a smooth rotation, but usually consist of a series of small steps (en-bloc turning). Parkinsonian patients may have difficulty getting started walking, but once started may actually walk faster and faster and be unable to stop (festination).

Steppage gait is associated with a foot drop, and this involves simply stepping higher with the affected leg so that the foot, which is hanging down, can clear the ground. These patients often give a history of stumbling/tripping over their toes on the weak side.

Scissor gait is seen in patients with a spastic paraparesis (spinal cord injury, cerebral palsy) and shows increased tone in the thigh adductors, such that whenever a step forward is attempted, the legs actually cross (hence the name scissor).

Sensory Examination

It is not necessary to memorize every possible combination of peripheral nerve or dermatomal sensory loss; however, some general guidelines are helpful. A pin (or a toothpick) is more accurate than a finger at mapping out areas of sensory loss.

Dermatomes to Remember

Root	Sensory Distribution
C6	Thumb
C7	Middle finger
C8	Pinky
T4	Nipple
T10	Umbilicus
L5	Big toe
S1	Sole of foot

Peripheral Nerves to Remember

Nerve	Sensory Distribution
Radial	Dorsum of hand
Ulnar	Pinky side of hand
Median	Palm of hand
Lateral femoral cutaneous	Lateral aspect of thigh
Peroneal	Lateral aspect of leg and dorsum of foot

If spinal cord compression is suspected, be certain to check for a **sensory level** on the trunk. **Perianal sensation** is important to check in patients with suspected cauda equina lesions.

Dissociated sensory loss, i.e., loss of pain and temperature on one side of the body and loss of vibration and proprioception on the other, is characteristic of a hemi-spinal lesion ipsilateral to the vibratory/proprioceptive loss (Brown-Sequard syndrome).

Deep Tendon Reflexes

An easy way to remember roughly which nerve roots serve which tendon reflexes is to start at the ankles and move up:

Count	Reflex	Root
1–2	Ankle	S1–S2
3–4	Knee	L3–L4
5–6	Biceps	C5–C6
7–8	Triceps	C7–C8

Grading of reflexes is as follows:

0	Absent
trace	Flicker of muscle contraction
1+	Hypoactive (may be normal, especially in muscular or obese patients)
2+	Normal
3+	Hyperactive, usually shows spread of reflex (may be normal, especially in thin or anxious patients)
4+	Hyperactive, clonus (always abnormal)

Spread of a reflex refers to when one reflex is being checked and muscle contraction occurs in another reflex. **Clonus** refers to repetitive reflex contractions after a single stimulus (usually elicited by abrupt dorsiflexion of the ankle by the examiner).

Plantar response is elicited by a quick, noxious stimulus (scratching with a key or other implement) to the lateral plantar aspect of the foot. A flexor response is when the great toe flexes and is the normal response of adults and older children. An extensor response (positive Babinski) is when the great toe extends (dorsiflexes) and the other toes spread apart. This is usually a sign of upper motor neuron disease (cerebral infarct, spinal cord compression, tumor), but can be normal in infants.

Neurologic Examination Summary

Mental Status
- Level of arousal: description
- Orientation: to self, place, time, situation
- Attention: digit span (normal 5–7)
- Speech: fluent? comprehension?

Cranial Nerves

- II—visual fields; consensual pupillary response
- III, IV, VI—pupillary reactivity/anisocoria; extraocular movements.
  doll's eyes—positive=eyes deviate in opposite direction of head turn.
  cold calorics—positive=eyes deviate tonically toward irrigated ear;
  with or without nystagmus away from irrigated ear.
- V—facial sensation; corneal reflex (sensory)—eyeblink when cornea touched with cotton wisp.
- VII—facial expression—if forehead movement is spared, lesion is above the facial nucleus (central); if forehead is weak, lesion is peripheral (Bell's palsy).
- VIII—hearing
- IX, X—palate symmetry, gag
- XI—head turn (sternocleidomastoid); shoulder shrug (trapezius)
- XII—tongue protrusion—deviates toward weak side

Motor Exam

- Bulk: check for symmetry; atrophy, fasciculations
- Tone: check for symmetry; is tone flaccid, spastic, rigid (cogwheeling)?
- Strength/power:
0	No movement
1	Trace/flicker of movement
2	Movement but not against gravity
3	Movement against gravity but not against resistance
4	Movement against partial resistance
5	Movement against full resistance
- Functional tests: Pronator drift—arms outstretched with palms up. Also, can patient rise from chair without pushing up with arms? stand on tiptoes? stand on heels? hop? hop on one foot?
- Tremor: resting tremor, postural or essential tremor

Cerebellar Examination

- Rapid alternation movements (dysdiadochokinesis)
- Finger-nose-finger (intention tremor)
- Heel-knee-shin.

Gait and Stance Examination

- Casual gait: observe as patient walks into room and during formal neuro exam
- Tandem gait: walk straight line heel to toe.
- Specific Gaits: ataxic—lurching, unsteady, swaying, wide stance; hemiparetic—decreased movement on weak side, circumduction of leg, decreased arm swing; parkinsonian—stooped, shuffling, retropulsion, en-bloc turns, festination; steppage—foot drop, walks with high step on weak foot; scissor—legs cross when stepping forward.

Sensory Examination

- Modalities to test: light touch, pinprick, temperature; vibration, proprioception.
- Sensory level: check with pin up and down trunk when suspicious of spinal cord lesion.

- Perianal sensation: check with suspicion of lower cord or cauda equina lesion

Deep Tendon Reflexes

• Root	• Reflex	• Grading of Reflexes	
S1–S2	Ankle	0	Absent
L3–L4	Knee	trace	Flicker of muscle contraction
C5–C6	Biceps	1+	Hypoactive
C7–C8	Triceps	2+	Normal
		3+	Hyperactive; may show spread
		4+	Hyperactive; pathologic; clonus

Clinical Symptoms and Signs

ALTERED MENTAL STATUS

I WATCH DEATH

Infection

Withdrawal
Acute metabolic derangement
Trauma
CNS pathology
Hypoxia

Deficiency
Endocrine
Acute vascular
Toxins/drugs
Heavy metals

CT, LP, AND EEG HIM

Cerebrovascular accident (brainstem ischemia/infarct)
Trauma

Low blood pressure/hypotension
Psychiatric

Anoxia/hypoxia
Neoplasm
Drugs/toxins/withdrawal

Epilepsy (nonconvulsive status, post-ictal)
Elevated blood pressure (hypertensive encephalopathy)
Glucose lack/hypoglycemia

Hemorrhage/bleed (intracranial, especially posterior fossa)
Infection (meningitis/encephalitis/sepsis)
Metabolic/endocrine

The first mnemonic is shorter but less comprehensive. The second mnemonic is more complete, and it pokes fun at a nonspecific approach to these patients. The CT, LP, and EEG are *not* required for all patients. The following describes an organized approach to this common problem.

Notes

Altered mental status refers to any acute or subacute change in the level of consciousness, ranging from mild confusion to deep coma. Chronic problems such as dementia or mental retardation are not considered in this discussion.

1. Initial treatment of *coma* or *unconsciousness* is aimed at rapidly identifying and treating any reversible process. **Protocol:**

   a. ABC's (Airway, Breathing, Circulation), vital signs, supplemental O_2 if necessary, pulse oximetry and ABG, ECG.

   b. IV line with normal saline. Send blood for CBC with differential and platelets, electrolytes, BUN, creatine, glucose, Ca, Mg, PT, PTT. Other tests to be considered include toxicology screen, liver enzymes, ammonia, blood cultures, urinalysis.

   - Fingerstick glucose, then 100 mg thiamine, then 50 ml 50% dextrose solution IV.
   - Rapid assessment of clinical situation, examination. Consider head CT scan. Emergent treatments include the following:

If opiate overdose suspected, Naloxone 0.01 mg/kg IV.

If seizure activity noted, Larazepam 2 mg IV.

If infection suspected, begin IV antibiotics, then proceed quickly with CT and LP.

If herniation detected, intubate, hyperventilate, mannitol 1 g/kg IV, CT, call neurosurgery.

- Definitive treatment will depend on the cause of the coma.

2. The examination of the comatose patient can be both quick and helpful in determining the etiology of the coma (see "How To Do a Good Neurologic Examination," page 207).

a. **Mental status:** Use specific descriptive terms; avoid vague terms like "sleepy" or "lethargic." To what level of stimulus does the patient respond? verbal, touch, pain?

b. **Cranial nerves:** Check pupils, eye movements (doll's eyes), corneals, facial symmetry, and gag (see page 209 for specifics on how to perform these tests). Cranial nerve abnormalities suggest brainstem dysfunction.

c. **Motor/sensory:** Observe the patient's movements. Note any obvious asymmetries. Passively move the patient's limbs to assess for asymmetry of muscle tone. Does the patient move spontaneously? Is the movement purposeful? Does the patient move to command? Does the patient move to noxious stimuli? When assessing the patient's reaction to noxious stimuli, note what sort of motor response is obtained. *Purposeful withdrawal* means moving the limb away from the stimulus and implies integrity of the cerebral cortex. *Decorticate posturing* is described as a flexion response in the upper extremity and extension in the lower, and suggests cortical dysfunction. *Decerebrate posturing* involves extension of both upper and lower extremities in response to a noxious stimulus, and this implies brainstem dysfunction. *No motor response* suggests severe brainstem dysfunction or peripheral paralysis (Guillain-Barré syndrome, iatrogenic paralysis).

d. **Reflexes:** Look for asymmetry of deep tendon reflexes. Check for clonus and Babinski responses.

3. There are three mechanisms of coma/depressed mental status.

a. Bilateral cerebral hemisphere dysfunction (e.g., bilateral infarcts, bilateral subdurals, hydrocephalus, meningitis, subarachnoid hemorrhage, generalized seizure activity)

b. Brainstem dysfunction only
- Direct brainstem injury (brainstem infarction, tumors or bleeds)
- Brainstem compression/displacement by supratentorial lesion (herniation secondary to supratentorial tumor, edema or bleed)

c. Diffuse cerebral and brainstem dysfunction (e.g., hypoxia, hypoglycemia, drug intoxications, uremia, hepatic encephalopathy, meningitis, subarachnoid hemorrhage)

Unilateral cerebral dysfunction alone does not cause coma (i.e., a unilateral infarct or tumor does not explain coma, unless herniation and compression of brainstem structures has occurred.

4. Approach to the differential diagnosis of coma:

Be aware that brainstem lesions do not always show up clearly on CT scans, so if brainstem pathology is strongly suspected and the CT scan is "normal," consider neurologic consultation and MRI scanning.

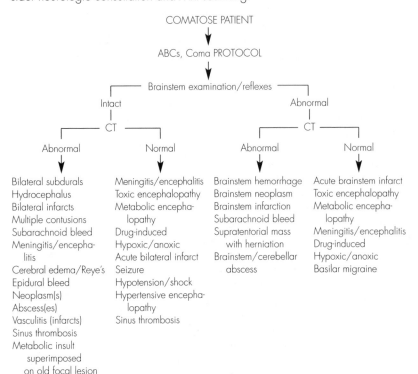

ATAXIA

<u>C</u>an't <u>S</u>tand <u>V</u>ery <u>W</u>ell

Cerebellar ataxia
Sensory ataxia
Vestibular ataxia
Weakness

Acute Ataxia

UNABLE TO STAND

Underlying weakness (may mimic ataxia)
Nutritional neuropathy (vitamin B_{12} deficiency)
Arteritis/vasculitis
Basilar migraine
Labyrinthitis/vestibular neuronitis
Encephalitis/infection

Trauma (postconcussive)
Other (rare metabolic or genetic diseases)

Stroke (ischemia or hemorrhage)
Toxins (drugs, toluene, mercury)
Alcohol intoxication
Neoplasm/paraneoplastic syndromes
Demyelination (Miller Fisher, Guillain Barré, MS)

Chronic Ataxia

CAN'T STAND

Congenital malformation/Chiari
Autosomal recessive ataxias
Nutritional (vitamin B_{12} deficiency)
Trauma (postconcussive)

Stroke sequelae
Toxins (drugs, toluene, alcohol)
Autosomal dominant ataxias
Neoplasm/paraneoplastic syndromes
Demyelination (MS)

Notes

Ataxia is the subjective complaint or objective finding of impaired coordination, usually manifested as an impairment of gait or dexterity in the absence of significant muscular weakness.

Dysdiadochokinesis is an impairment of the ability to perform rapid alternating movements.

Dysmetria is impairment in the normal acceleration and deceleration of directed movements. Usually evaluated by finger-nose-finger and heel-knee-shin tests.

Intention tremor is an exaggerated oscillation of a limb, most pronounced as it is approaching a target, and essentially absent at rest or at the beginning of a movement. Intention tremor is a manifestation of dysmetria.

Titubation is a moderate frequency head tremor, usually anteroposterior.

1. The **time course** of ataxia helps narrow the differential diagnosis. Acute ataxias usually are due to acute brain injury (trauma, infarct, bleed), intoxication, infection, inflammation/autoimmune reactions (vasculitis, paraneoplastic), or migraine. Chronic ataxias usually are caused by congenital malformations, sequelae of brain injury (post-stroke, cerebral palsy, trauma), multiple sclerosis, brain tumors, or genetic diseases (Friedreich's, ataxia-telangiectasia).

2. **Evaluation** of ataxia includes coordination testing and sensory testing.

   a. Finger-nose-finger: The patient is asked to use the index finger to alternately touch his/her nose and the examiner's outstretched finger.

   b. Heel-knee-shin: The patient is asked to touch one heel to the opposite knee and then move the heel down the shin to the foot.

   c. Rapid alternating movements: The patient is to alternately pronate and supinate either hand, usually patting on the thigh or another horizontal surface. In the lower extremities, this may be tested by having the patient tap either foot on the floor.

   d. Proprioception: Position sense is tested by having the patient identify whether a digit is being moved up or down at a joint (usually interphalangeal finger or toe) with the eyes closed. At least one joint on each limb is tested several times. If a deficit is detected distally, continue testing proximally until the patient is able to identify movements correctly (i.e., if position sense is impaired in the fingers, follow with testing at the wrist, elbow or even shoulder to determine the extent of the deficit).

   e. Romberg sign: This is tested by having the patient assume a comfortable stance with the eyes open and the feet as close as possible, then closing his/her eyes. Continued stability is a negative Romberg, and instability/falling with eyes closed is a positive Romberg. A positive Romberg is indicative of impaired proprioceptive input. *Romberg testing is not useful in patients unable to stand steadily with their eyes open.*

3. Ataxia may be divided into four categories that often can be distinguished by careful history and examination. Some disorders may be associated with more than one type of ataxia (in particular, cerebellar and vestibular ataxia often occur together).

   a. **Cerebellar ataxia** is characterized by dysmetria, dysdiadochokinesis, hypotonia, and unsteady gait in the absence of significant motor weakness, nausea, or vomiting. Nystagmus may be present. Cerebellar ataxia may be unilateral or bilateral. Unilateral cerebellar ataxia suggests a focal lesion (*tumor, infarct, bleed, multiple sclerosis*), while bilateral cerebellar ataxia is more likely due to diffuse causes (*alcohol, drug intoxication, paraneoplastic*).

   b. **Sensory ataxia** is caused by impaired position sense and not by cerebellar pathology. Findings consistent with sensory ataxia include impaired sensation, particularly proprioception and vibration. Nausea, vomiting, and nystagmus are not seen with sensory ataxia. Etiologies include neuropathies and spinal cord dorsal column pathology (e.g., *vitamin B_{12} deficiency, neurosyphilis/tabes dorsalis*).

   c. **Vestibular ataxia** typically is associated with vertigo, nausea and vomiting. Impaired coordination, diminished hearing, nystagmus, and gait instability also may occur. Vestibular causes of ataxia include *labyrinthitis/vestibular neuronitis, brainstem ischemia,* and *multiple sclerosis,* among others.

   d. **Weakness** due to hemiparesis may manifest by falling or gait disturbance and is not true ataxia. In the setting of significant motor weakness, it is difficult to assess coordination separately. Significant focal weakness should raise the possibility of a focal cerebral lesion (*tumor, infarct, bleed, abscess*).

4. Intoxication is a common cause of acute ataxia. Offending agents include many anticonvulsants (e.g., phenytoin, carbamazepine) and alcohol.

5. A good **family history** is essential in the evaluation of chronic or recurrent ataxia. Migraines often occur in persons with a positive family history of migraine headaches (aura, photophobia, nausea, vomiting). Metabolic diseases presenting with recurrent or progressive ataxia often have autosomal recessive inheritance (maple syrup urine disease, ataxia telangiectasia, Friedreich ataxia). Autosomal dominant forms of ataxia include von Hippel-Lindau disease (cerebellar hemangioblastoma), olivopontocerebellar atrophy, and Machado-Joseph disease.

6. Work-up for ataxia depends on the differential diagnosis. Neuroimaging (CT acutely, but MRI is better for chronic symptoms) is necessary if a focal lesion is suspected. Acute, nonfocal ataxia warrants testing for alcohol and drug intoxication. In patients with known malignancy, work-up for metastases (CT/MRI) and paraneoplastic syndromes (autoantibodies) should be considered. Lumbar puncture should be performed in cases where CNS infection is likely (fever, meningismus). Patients with primarily sensory ataxia should be evaluated for causes of sensory neuropathy and dorsal column pathology by checking VDRL/RPR, glucose, and vitamin B_{12}.

Autonomic Disorders

A BP DROP, I GUESS

Amyloidosis

Botulism
Parkinson's disease

Diabetes
Riley-Day syndrome/familial dysautonomia
Oncologic/paraneoplastic
Porphyria

Idiopathic/**I**atrogenic

Guillain-Barré syndrome
Uremia
Ethanol/alcoholism
Shy-Drager syndrome
Spinal cord disorders

Notes

Autonomic disorders constitute a wide range of neurologic derangements, which manifest primarily through symptoms of autonomic dysfunction, including but not limited to orthostatic hypotension/syncope, cardiac arrhythmias, altered lacrimation, impaired temperature regulation, diaphoresis/anhidrosis, sexual dysfunction, and bowel/bladder problems.

1. Autonomic dysfunction can occur due to impairment of the autonomic nervous system in the brain (*Shy-Drager syndrome, hypothalamic tumor, Parkinson's disease*), spinal cord (*tumor, myelitis, multiple sclerosis*), autonomic nerves (*diabetes, Guillain-Barré syndrome, amyloidosis*) or neuromuscular junction (*botulism*). Systemic diseases (*peripheral vascular disease, connective tissue disease, prostatism*) may manifest with autonomic symptoms. Autonomic impairment becomes more pronounced with advancing age, prolonged bedrest, and various medications.
2. Autonomic symptoms are rarely the sole manifestation of an underlying illness, and the diagnosis often is made based on the **combination of autonomic**

impairment and other cardinal signs/symptoms. For example, the following diagnoses feature autonomic symptoms in combination with others:

    a. *Parkinson's, Shy-Drager*—bradykinesia, rigidity, postural instability (resting tremor in Parkinsons)

    b. *Guillain Barré*—subacute onset, ascending paralysis, areflexia, autonomic instability

    c. *Peripheral vascular disease, diabetes*—orthostatic hypotension, impaired distal circulation, poor wound healing in extremities (hyperglycemia in *diabetes*).

3. Management of autonomic disorders often is symptomatic, *once the underlying condition has been diagnosed and is being treated.*

    a. Orthostatic hypotension—maintain good hydration and sodium, gradual postural changes, discontinue hypotension medications, avoid prolonged inactivity. Fluorohydrocortisone may be helpful in patients with difficult to control orthostasis.

    b. Bladder dysfunction—flaccid bladders may respond to bethanechol. Spastic bladders may be relaxed using propantheline and/or oxybutynin. Intermittent self-catheterization often is helpful in preventing urinary incontinence in certain patients (*multiple sclerosis, spinal cord disease*).

    c. Sexual dysfunction—penile implant, medication, endocrine and urologic/gynecologic evaluation.

DIPLOPIA

HINT: IS CT DONE?

Central
Hemorrhage, cerebellar
Infarct/TIA
Neoplasm (brainstem tumor)
Toxic/metabolic

Peripheral
Infectious/meningitis
Subarachnoid hemorrhage/aneurysm

Cancer (carcinomatous meningitis, cavernous tumor)
Thyroid ophthalmopathy

Diabetes
Orbital process (orbital fracture/mass)
Neuromuscular junction disease (myasthenia)
Eye problem (lens subluxation)

CT WHOM? MOST CT IMAGED

Central
CVA/ischemia, brainstem
Toxins/drugs

Wernicke's
Hemorrhage, cerebellar
Oncologic (brainstem tumor)
Multiple sclerosis

Peripheral
Myasthenia gravis
Orbital process (orbital fracture/mass)
Subarachnoid hemorrhage
Trauma (shearing injury to cranial nerve)

Cavernous sinus process
Thyroid ophthalmopathy

Infections (herpes zoster ophthalmicus)
Malignancy (carcinomatous meningitis)
Aneurysmal compression
Granulomatous (sarcoid, Tolosa-Hunt)
Eye problem (lens subluxation)
Diabetes

Also under Peripheral: increased intracranial pressure (as in pseudotumor cerebri) can cause cranial nerve (CN) VI palsy with resultant diplopia.

Notes

Diplopia is the subjective symptom of double vision.
   Dysconjugate gaze is the objective examination finding of eye misalignment, which may or may not be associated with symptoms of diplopia.

1. Examination includes direct observation of eye movements in all axes of movement. Does the patient report resolution of diplopia if one eye is covered? Is the visual acuity in both eyes equal?

2. Drugs and toxins are a common cause of diplopia. Offending agents include carbamazepine, phenytoin, and alcohol.

3. Congenital strabismus, if not corrected, leads to suppression of the visual image from one eye. Thus, it is possible for a patient with obviously dysconjugate gaze *not* to complain of diplopia.

4. Monocular diplopia (diplopia with one eye covered) almost always is secondary to intraocular disease.

5. A **CN III palsy** may be a cause of diplopia. A complete CN III palsy causes ptosis; inability to move the eye up, down, or inward; and a dilated, unreactive pupil. Many are incomplete. Compressive lesions of CN III (aneurysms, tumors) are most likely to cause pupillary involvement and should be imaged. A patient with appropriate impairment of eye movement and no pupillary involvement most likely has a **medical CN III palsy** (presumed to be a microinfarction of the nerve fibers), especially if the patient has diabetes. Generally these patients do not need a brain CT, and palsy resolves over a few weeks. They should be followed closely, however, to ensure that the pupil does not become involved.

6. Diplopia can be a manifestation of **cavernous sinus disease**. The cavernous sinus is an intracranial compartment located behind the orbit and lateral to the pituitary. The carotid artery, CNs III, IV, and VI, and the V1 branch of V pass through this area. The V2 branch of CN V occupies the most inferior portion of the cavernous sinus. Whenever a combination of CN deficits involving III, IV, V1, V2, and/or VI is detected, a structural lesion in the cavernous sinus should be ruled out with an imaging study, preferentially a gadolinium-enhanced MRI.

7. **Herniation** is a condition where a supratentorial mass causes lateral displacement of the brainstem and can cause an ipsilateral palsy involving the pupil. Patients who are herniating have altered mental status, and thus are not likely to be complaining of anything, let alone diplopia. The typical clinical picture in which herniation is a concern is the comatose patient with a "blown" (i.e., fixed and dilated) pupil. Herniation requires immediate treatment to reduce intracranial pressure (hyperventilation, mannitol) and prompt CT scanning to determine the cause of the problem. *Patients with a dilated pupil and a normal mental status are not herniating.*

8. Central causes of diplopia listed above involve primarily the brainstem and cerebellum. There may be other evidence of brainstem or cerebellar dysfunction (other CN palsies, ataxia, hyperreflexia, upgoing toes, hemiparesis). *Imaging studies are indicated in patients with other focal neurologic findings.*

9. Peripheral causes of diplopia listed above involve the eye itself and cranial nerves (III, IV, VI). A careful ophthalmologic examination is warranted, particularly in cases of monocular diplopia. *Imaging studies of the brain generally are not needed for intraocular causes of diplopia, medical CN III palsy, or myasthenia gravis.* However, when uncertain about exam findings, imaging may help to eliminate the more ominous possibilities.

DIZZINESS

So Very Dizzy Now

Syncope/presyncope
Vertigo
Disequilibrium
Nonspecific

OLD SPINNING MAMA

Otolith (benign positional vertigo)
Low blood sugar
Demyelination (multiple sclerosis)

Stroke/TIA/bleed
Post-traumatic
Intravascular volume depletion/hypotension
Neuroma/neoplasm
Neuronitis/labyrinthitis
Intoxication (EtOH, drugs, medications)
Neuropathy/myelopathy
GI bleed/anemia

Multifactorial/migraine
Aminoglycosides/ototoxic medications
Meniere's disease
Anxiety/hyperventilation

A HOBBLED MAN SPINS

Anemia

Hyperventilation/psychiatric
Other (multifactorial, migraine)
Benign positional vertigo
Bleed/hemorrhage
Labyrinthitis/vestibular neuronitis
Endocrine/metabolic (hypoglycemia)
Demyelination (multiple sclerosis)

Meniere's disease
Aminoglycoside toxicity
Neuropathy/myelopathy

Syncope/hypotension
Post-traumatic
Intoxication (EtOH, drugs, medication)
Neuroma/neoplasm
Stroke/TIA

Notes

1. A complaint of dizziness may mean different things to different people. Try to historically determine which category of symptoms the patient has (these categories can be remembered by the mnemonic "So Very Dizzy Now."

   a. **Syncope/presyncope:** Lightheadedness, faintness, postural. DDx more likely to include arrhythmia, decreased cardiac output, orthostasis, autonomic neuropathy, vasovagal reflex.

   b. **Vertigo:** Illusion of movement of patient or surroundings, often with nausea, vomiting. DDx more likely to include benign positional vertigo, labyrinthitis, Meniere's, MS, post-traumatic, vestibular nerve neuroma.

   c. **Disequilibirum:** unsteadiness, feeling "drunk," clumsiness, wobbly. DDx more likely to include drug intoxication, EtOH, aminoglycoside ototoxicity, severe peripheral neuropathy, multifactorial.

   d. **Nonspecific:** Anxiety, weakness, vague, difficult to describe. DDx more likely to include hyperventilation, systemic disease (anemia, metabolic), multifactorial.

2. When examining a patient with dizziness, try to reproduce the patient's symptoms with a variety of maneuvers.

    a. Check for orthostasis by blood pressure and pulse (supine and standing) and note any subjective complaints the patient has.

    b. Perform the Hall-Pike (Barany) maneuver (see 6.a.) to diagnose benign positional vertigo.

    c. Hyperventilation may reproduce symptoms of dizziness associated with anxiety or panic attacks.

    d. Valsalva maneuver may reproduce symptoms related to decreased cardiac output.

A patient may complain of some form of dizziness with more than one of these maneuvers. It is most helpful if the patient can determine which maneuver actually reproduces the symptoms comprising the chief complaint.

3. Vertebrobasilar ischemia *rarely causes isolated vertigo.* Investigate thoroughly for other evidence of brainstem/cerebellar dysfunction (other cranial nerve palsies, ataxia, hyperreflexia, upgoing toes, hemiparesis).

4. *Meniere's disease* is associated with hearing loss. *Benign positional vertigo* and *labyrinthitis/vestibular neuronitis* are not.

5. In many cases of dizziness, no single factor stands out as the causative one. A combination of factors may conspire to make the patient more symptomatic than any one factor would alone. For example, a patient may have mild *diabetic neuropathy, cataracts,* and a history of *alcohol abuse.* The combination of peripheral neuropathy, decreased visual acuity, and diminished cerebellar function, plus the possibility of a diabetic autonomic neuropathy, put this patient in the multifactorial category of this differential diagnosis.

6. *Benign positional vertigo (BPV)* is characterized by attacks of vertigo following a change in head position, most commonly rolling over in bed or looking up. It is most common in the elderly and is thought to be caused by free-floating calcifications (otoliths) in the posterior semicircular canal.

    a. The **Hallpike maneuver** is used to diagnose this condition. The starting position is with the patient sitting, the examiner standing to the side, and facing the patient, with the examiner's hands supporting the patient's head. The patient may hold onto the examiner's elbow. The final position is with the patient supine, eyes open, the neck extended 30° below the plane of the bed, and the head rotated 30° laterally toward the side being tested (the side the examiner is on). The maneuver involves rapidly moving the patient from the first position to the second. The test is considered positive (diagnostic for benign positional vertigo) if, after a brief latency of 3–30 seconds, the patient develops a torsional nystagmus in the direction of the side being tested. Upon sitting up, there often is a torsional nystagmus in the opposite direction. Each side is tested to determine which side is involved. Occasionally, both sides are affected.

    b. **Torsional nystagmus** is the hallmark of BPV. The eye on the side of the affected labyrinth demonstrates a mostly lateral nystagmus toward the affected side, while the opposite eye shows a more rotatory component, with the top of the globe rotating toward the affected side.

c. A variation of the Hallpike known as **Epley's maneuver** may be used to dislodge the offending calcification. The Hallpike is performed to the symptomatic side, then, without allowing the patient to sit up, the patient is rolled to the asymptomatic side into a lateral decubitus position. Finally, from this lateral decubitus position, the patient is allowed to sit up. The patient should feel vertiginous throughout the maneuver, burt after it is completed, the vertigo should resolve.

d. If Epley's maneuver is unsuccessful, the patient can be instructed in vestibular exercises to desensitize the vestibular apparatus. These consist of self-administered Hallpike maneuvers done two to three times a day, with five repetitions each time.

e. Vestibular suppressants such as meclizine prolong the period of vestibular desensitization and are generally less helpful, except in severe cases involving dehydration risk from nausea and vomiting.

HEADACHE

CT SCAN ME?

Cluster
Tension

Sinusitis/otitis/mastoiditis
Craving (drug-seeking vs. rebound)
Aneurysm/arteritis
Neuralgia, trigeminal

Migraine
Elevated intracranial pressure (subdural hematoma, hemorrhage, AVM, tumor, pseudotumor, hypertension, hydrocephalus)

Also: infection (meningitis/meningoencephalitis), metabolic, psychiatric, post-LP, osteoarthritis, post-concussive, sinus thrombosis

CAN'T STOP HEAD PAINS

Cluster/migraine
Arteritis (temporal, lupus)
Neuralgia (trigeminal)
Tension headache

Sinus thrombosis (venous)
Trauma (post-concussive)
Osteoarthritis/musculoskeletal
Post-LP

Hydrocephalus
Elevated blood pressure
Aneurysm/subarachnoid hemorrhage
Drugs (opiate rebound headache, steroid withdrawal, oral contraceptives)

Pseudotumor cerebri
Arteriovenous malformation
Infections (meningitis/meningoencephalitis)
Neoplasm
Sinusitis/otitis/mastoiditis

Also: psychiatric, metabolic (hyperthyroid, Cushing's, chronic lung disease with hypercapnia)

Notes

Headache is a general term used to describe any painful sensation involving the structures of the cranium, face, and/or neck.

1. History is all-important in the diagnosis of headache. Questions to ask include the following:
    a. Precipitating factors—stress, trauma, certain foods, caffeine, alcohol, time of day, drug use
    b. Prodromal symptoms—visual scotoma, focal weakness/numbness, aphasia
    c. Rapidity of onset—seconds, minutes, hours
    d. Location (uni- or bilateral, temporal, occipital, cervical) and nature (throbbing, stabbing, pressure-like, lancinating) of pain
    e. Associated symptoms—nausea, diplopia, vertigo, vomiting, lacrimation,

fever, gait disturbance, altered mental status, seizures, photophobia, exacerbated by standing

  f. Duration—seconds, minutes, hours, days, daily/chronic

  g. Alleviating factors—quiet, sleep, analgesics, darkness, prescription medications

  h. Other pertinent medical history—cancer, hypertension, pregnancy, history of similar headaches, family history of migraine, medications, trauma

2. To scan or not to scan? Worrisome complaints such as **new-onset severe headache, seizures, recent change in pattern of a chronic headache, and/or focal neurologic deficits** may indicate the need for an imaging study. However, routine scanning of patients with symptoms of classic migraine and a nonfocal neurologic exam has a very low yield of revealing a treatable intracranial abnormality. Routine scanning of patients with chronic headache complaints (migraine or nonmigraine) and a nonfocal neurologic exam also tends to have a low yield of demonstrating treatable intracranial disease.

3. Approach to diagnosis of chronic headache: see table. Be aware of types of chronic headaches that don't fit well into these categories, including temporal arteritis, lupus, some pituitary tumors, cluster headaches, hypercapnea secondary to pulmonary disease, and some endocrinopathies.

Approach to Diagnosis of Chronic Headache

| Characteristics | Headache Type | | |
	Migraine	*Tension*	*Elevated ICP*
Onset	Minutes	Hours–days	Days–weeks
Time course of pain	Maximal in 15–60 minutes, **normal between headaches**	Moderate, **waxing and waning, may be persistent**	**Gradually worsening** over time
Duration Hours–(days)	Hours–weeks–	(Days)–weeks–(months)	months
Location	Unilateral, but can be on either side	Bilateral, esp. frontal, occipital	Unilateral if focal lesion, otherwise bilateral
Quality of pain	Throbbing, pulsatile	Achey, pressure-like, muscle tension	Pressure-like, dull
Nausea, vomiting	**Common with headache**	No	Nocturnal, **early morning**
Light and noise sensitivity	Common	No	No

(Table continued on next page.)

Approach to Diagnosis of Chronic Headache *(Continued)*

Characteristics	Headache Type		
	Migraine	*Tension*	*Elevated ICP*
Focal neurologic signs	**Stereotyped and transient**, often visual (scotoma)	No	Gradual onset and progressive, sometimes diplopia
Seizures	Very rare	No	Occasional
Papilledema	No	No	Yes

4. Summary of specific headache types:

Type	Symptoms
Cluster	Unilateral stabbing peri/retro-orbital pain; ipsilateral lacrimation, rhinorrhea Occurs in "clusters" of daily attacks over a period of weeks, between clusters may be asymptomatic for weeks/months/years Duration usually 15–30 minutes, may last 2–3 hours Unlike migraine patients, may be agitated, generally do not sit still
Migraine, common	Episodic, recurrent, throbbing, uni- or bilateral pain Associated with light and noise sensitivity, nausea and vomiting Duration usually 2–4 hours, may last up to 2–4 days Patients seek quiet, dark areas and try to sleep and be still
Migraine, classic	Similar to common migraine but preceded by focal neurologic disturbance (visual scotoma, numbness, aphasia, vertigo) and lasting a few minutes to an hour
Temporal arteritis	Throbbing temporal or bitemporal pain in elderly patient Associated with monocular visual loss, jaw claudication, tender temporal artery(ies) to palpation
Increased intracranial pressure With focal lesion Without focal lesion	Wakens from sleep Associated with early morning vomiting May have papilledema on funduscopic examination • Tumor—focal neurologic deficit, seizures, h/o systemic cancer • Abscess—focal neurologic deficit, seizures, may have fever, evidence of systemic emboli (check fundi, nailbeds, cardiac murmur) • AVM—focal neurologic deficit, seizures, head bruit • Pseudotumor cerebri—may have visual loss (decreased visual fields and/or decreased visual acuity), sixth nerve palsy/diplopia • Hydrocephalus—may have gait disturbance, decreased upgaze, incontinence
Post-LP	Often positional, better when lying down Duration may last up to a week

(Table continued on next page.)

Type	Symptoms
Subarachnoid hemorrhage	Abrupt onset, may have initial loss of consciousness "Worst headache of my life" May have fever, stiff neck, altered mental status
Meningitis/ encephalitis	Associated with fever, stiff neck, altered mental status May have seizures (especially herpes encephalitis)
Tension	"Pressure-like" or "hat-band" bifrontal or bioccipital pain May be associated with neck/shoulder/back pain Often chronic
Rebound	Associated with worsening of headache as analgesics/narcotics wear off Diagnosis of exclusion

5. Therapy for headache is dependent on the diagnosis. Treatment with analgesics/narcotics may temporarily alleviate discomfort, but does not treat the cause of the headache. **In general, beware of treating pain while leaving the underlying etiology untreated** (e.g., meningitis, hemorrhage).

LOSS OF CONSCIOUSNESS

VAGAL SYNCOPE

Volume loss/bleeding
Aortic dissection
Glucose drop
Autonomic dysfunction
Low cardiac output

Seizure
Your mama's visiting/anxiety/psychogenic
Neurocardiogenic/reflex
CVA/subarachnoid hemorrhage
Orthostatic hypotension
Pulmonary embolism/peripheral vascular disease
Elevated blood pressure

Also: basilar migraine

ACLS! I HAVE TO PASS OUT

Aortic aneurysm/dissection
Cough/micturition/reflex syncope
Low glucose
Sinus hypersensitivity, carotid

Iatrogenic/drug/medication

Hemorrhage, subarachnoid
Autonomic neuropathy
Vasovagal syncope
Ethanol intoxication

Transient ischemic attack
Orthostatic hypotension (hypovolemia, poor vascular tone)

Psychogenic
Asystole/heart block
Seizure
Subclavian steal

Outflow obstruction
Underpowered heart/cardiomyopathy
Tachyarrhythmia

Also: basilar migraine

THIS MADE ME VAGAL

TIA/cerebral ischemia
Hypertension
Intracranial hemorrhage (subarachnoid)
Seizure

Myocardial infarction
Aortic dissection
Drugs/alcohol
Emotions/psychiatric

Migraine
Embolism, pulmonary

Volume loss
Arrhythmia
Glucose drop
Autonomic
Low cardiac output (congestive heart failure, aortic
    stenosis, pulmonary hypertension

Also: neurocardiogenic/reflex syncope

Notes

Syncope (i.e., fainting) is defined as a transient loss of consciousness and postural tone due to impaired cerebral blood flow.

1. A description of the spell is crucial to appropriate workup and diagnosis. The patient as well as any eyewitnesses should be questioned. Important historical information can be divided into three time periods:
    a. **Prior to the event**—postural changes (e.g., patient stands up), precipitating factors (skipped meals, physical exertion, severe stress, cough, micturition), symptoms (headache, dizziness, chest pain, shortness of breath, heart palpitation, faintness, focal neurologic symptoms, nausea), and eyewitness descriptions (altered behavior/mentation, pallor, excessive sweating).
    b. **During the event** (usually from the eyewitness)—rapidity of onset, duration of episode/unresponsiveness, involuntary motor activity, apnea, overt seizure activity, injury to the patient, loss of continence.
    c. **After the event**—orientation/responsiveness, amnesia, rapidity of recovery to baseline mental state, recurrent episodes.
In addition, pertinent information about pre-existing medical conditions, current medications, recent alcohol/drug ingestion, and family history of fainting or seizures should be sought.
2. Conditions that may mimic syncope include *seizure, drug/alcohol intoxication, subarachnoid hemorrhage* and *basilar migraine*. Conditions associated with faintness but in which complete loss of consciousness is rare include *hypoglycemia, anemia, hyperventilation, panic disorder,* and *hysteria*.
3. The differential for syncope can be thought of in four major categories:
    a. **Neurocardiogenic**—reflex inhibition of heart via autonomic nervous system
       • Includes vasovagal attack, carotid sinus syndrome, micturition, cough, valsalva, emotional stress.
       • Distinguished by the presence of precipitating event and absence of cardiac and peripheral vascular pathology. Usually in younger persons.

b. **Orthostatic**—drop in blood pressure due to inability to maintain vascular tone
- Medications, postural change, neuropathies (especially autonomic), neurodegenerative disease, peripheral vascular disease, hypovolemia.
- Distinguished by orthostatic tachycardia/hypotension on exam, and history of spells correlating with postural change.

c. **Cardiogenic**—direct cardiac pathology
- Cardiomyopathy, aortic valve disease, tachyarrhythmia, bradyarrhythmia/asystole.
- Distinguished by cardiac symptomatology (e.g., chest pain, palpitations), known cardiac disease, and ECG abnormalities during spell.

d. **Other**—miscellaneous
- Hypoglycemia, cerebral ischemia/infarct, intracranial hemorrhage, basilar migraine, drug/alcohol intoxication, pulmonary embolism (PE), aortic dissection.
- Systemic metabolic causes (hypoglycemia, intoxication) associated with "wooziness," more gradual onset. Vascular causes usually due to a sudden mechanical obstruction of cerebral vasculature (infarct, dissection). Catastrophic causes include PE and intracranial bleed.

4. Reflex syncope is due to excessive vagal stimulation, which slows the heart rate and decreases cerebral blood flow, causing unconsciousness. **Carotid sinus syndrome** is due to excessive pressure sensitivity of the carotid sinus. Tight collars or other external pressure on the neck can provoke syncope. Other known provocateurs of reflex syncope include micturition, valsalva maneuver, and coughing. **Vasovagal syncope** is a type of reflex syncope triggered by pain, fear, or other sudden emotional stress. It typically occurs in adolescents and young adults and may be more likely in the setting of prolonged standing, fatigue, and/or fasting.

5. Medications commonly implicated in orthostatic hypotension include antihypertensive drugs, diuretics, nitroglycerin and other arterial vasodilators, tricyclic antidepressants, phenothiazines, lithium, calcium channel blockers, and beta blockers.

6. Cardiac causes of syncope can be revealed by physical exam and ECG. It may be necessary to monitor patients with cardiac telemetry or a Holter monitor to detect a transient arrhythmia. Echocardiography may demonstrate **aortic valve disease** or **cardiomyopathy**.

7. Initial workup for a transient loss of consciousness is fairly straightforward:

a. ABCs; if episode over, then proceed with further evaluation including history and exam.

b. ECG and blood pressure monitors.

c. Accucheck, pulse oximetry.

d. Laboratory studies to be considered: electrolytes, glucose, BUN/Cr, CBC, ethanol, tox screen.

8. Further workup (and treatment) depends on the suspected cause of the episode.

a. Seizure: CT/MRI, EEG.

b. Cardiac: cardiac telemetry/Holter monitor, echocardiogram, cardiac enzymes

        Pulmonary embolism—VQ scan, pulmonary angiogram

c. Orthostatic: some cases may need provocative testing such as tilt table

d. Neurocardiogenic: if initial workup negative and history suggestive of reflex syncope, generally no further workup is required.

e. Cerebrovascular:

        Aortic dissection/aneurysm—chest x-ray/CT, angiogram

        Subarachnoid hemorrhage/cerebral aneurysm—head CT MRI, Angiogram, lumbar puncture

        Transient ischemic attack—head CT/MRI, carotic/vertebral doppler, angiogram, coagulation lab studies

f. Metabolic:

        Hypoglycemia—check serum glucose, administer IV glucose

        Intoxication—blood ethanol, serum or urine tox screen

MONOCULAR VISUAL LOSS

BLIND

Blood vessels (arteritis, hemorrhage, embolism)
Lens (cataract)
Infection
Nerve (tumor, optic neuritis, glaucoma—via pressure on nerve)
Detached retina/other retinal disease

GRAVE VISIONED

Glaucoma
Retinal/ocular migraine
Arteritis, temporal
Venous thrombosis (central retinal vein occlusion)
Embolism (central retinal artery occlusion)

Vascular occlusion (carotid)
Infections (CMV retinitis)
Senile cataract
Intraocular bleed
Optic neuritis
Neoplasm (optic nerve glioma)
Elevated serum vicosity (sickle cell, polycythemia)
Detached retina

MONO-VISIONED

Migraine, ocular/retinal
Occlusion, central retinal artery
Neoplasm
Occlusion, central retinal vein

Vasculitis, temporal (giant cell)
Infection
Senile cataracts
Intraocular bleed
Optic neuritis
Not monocular visual loss
Elevated serum viscosity
Detached retina

Also: glaucoma

Notes

Monocular visual loss is either a subjective report of transient visual loss in one eye (as opposed to one visual field) or an objective finding of decreased visual acuity in one eye. Pseudotumor cerebri and other causes of increased intracranial pressure generally produce bilateral signs/symptoms

1. **It is critical to distinguish between monocular visual loss and a visual field cut.** With monocular visual loss, visual acuity is diminished in *one eye*, and the lesion is in the eye or optic nerve. With a visual field cut, vision is impaired in a particular area of the visual field in *both eyes*, and the lesion is in the optic tract

or the brain. **This distinction can be made clear by testing visual acuity and visual fields one eye at a time.** Sometimes, patients mistake a visual field cut for monocular visual loss on the same side ("Doc, I can't see out of my left eye."). On exam, however, the patient demonstrates a left visual field cut in both eyes.

2. True monocular visual loss is caused by a lesion in the eye or optic nerve (anterior to the optic chiasm), and thus may be due to problems in the lens, retina, blood vessels, or the optic nerve itself.

3. **Amaurosis fugax** is the subjective complaint of transient visual loss in one eye, often described as a veil or shade coming over the eye. This is essentially a transient ischemic attack of the retina, and may be caused by emboli from the heart to the central retinal artery, an ulcerated carotid plaque causing emboli or occlusion, or temporal arteritis involving the carotid artery.

4. It is critical not to miss the diagnosis of **temporal arteritis** because prompt treatment could prevent complete infarction of the retina. The classic clinical picture is a person > age 65, with unilateral or bilateral severe headache, tender temporal arteries, low-grade fever, anemia, and elevated ESR. Amaurosis fugax, polymyalgia rheumatica, and jaw claudication may occur. Treatment is with prednisone 60–100 mg/d and should not be delayed to obtain temporal artery biopsy, but biopsy should be performed bilaterally within 3 days of initiating steroids. ESR should be monitored and used to guide therapy. In cases of acute retinal ischemia, IV methylprednisolone has been used.

5. Ophthalmoscopic examination is also of great importance in evaluating monocular visual loss, since central retinal artery occlusion, central retinal vein occlusion, retinal detachment, cataracts, infections/retinitis, hemorrhage, and optic disc edema can be detected.

PTOSIS

LID DROP

Lid infiltration (by tumor or inflammatory tissue)
Infection (zoster, botulism)
Diabetes/thyroid

Drugs
Receptor antibodies (myasthenia)
Oculosympathetic palsy/oculomotor palsy
Proptosis

TENSILON ME, DOC

Third nerve palsy
Eyedrops (steroid)
Neuromuscular junction disease (myasthenia)
Surgery
Infection (herpes zoster ophthalmicus)
Lid infiltration (by tumor or inflammatory tissue)
Oculosympathetic palsy (Horner's syndrome)
Neurotoxins (botulism)

Myopathy (muscular dystrophy, myotonic dystrophy)
Enophthalmos (eyeball retraction into orbit)

Diabetes/thyroid disease
Opposite lid retraction
Cluster headache

Also: congenital ptosis

Notes

Ptosis is a physical finding of one palpebral fissure being smaller than the other, i.e., a drooping eyelid.

1. Ptosis may be the result of a partial or complete third nerve palsy (with associated ophthalmoplegia and pupillary dilation/unreactivity). For a full description of third nerve palsy, see notes 5–9 under the heading Diplopia, page 225.
2. Ptosis is part of the oculosympathetic palsy or Horner's syndrome, which consists of **unilateral ptosis, miosis (small pupil)**, and **anhidrosis of the face (decreased sweating)**.

The sympathetic pathways go down the spinal cord to the thoracic level, where they exit the cord and ascend the neck as the sympathetic trunk to the superior cervical ganglion, then follow the internal carotid artery and, ultimately, the V1 division of cranial nerve V to the eye.

Any lesion that interrupts the oculosympathetic pathways can result in Horner's syndrome, including tumor (lung, mediastinal, thyroid, pharyngeal, lymphoma, spinal cord), trauma, and congenital causes, as well as (less likely) carotid dissection/occlusion, cervical disc or rib, meningitis, brainstem infarct, syrinx, polio, pneumothorax, and ALS. A significant proportion of Horner's cases are idiopathic, with a high frequently of diabetes and hypertension in this idiopathic group.

3. Neuromuscular disease, specifically myasthenia gravis, may present as ptosis (often bilateral but asymmetric). This often is associated with fluctuating ocular palsies (diplopia), facial weakness, weakness of speech and swallowing, and neck and shoulder girdle weakness. Not infrequently, the weakness affects the muscles of respiration. Characteristically, muscles are fatiguable if subjected to sustained contraction. Pupillary muscles, smooth muscle, cardiac muscle, and sensation are unaffected.

The **Tensilon (edrophonium) test** is helpful in the diagnosis of myasthenia. Myasthenia is caused by autoantibodies to the acetylcholine (ACh) receptor. Normally, ACh crosses the synapse, binds to the receptor, and eventually is metabolized by acethylcholine esterase (AChE). In myasthenia, the ACh receptor is partially blocked, and ACh is metabolized by AChE before it can bind the receptor. Edrophonium is an AChE inhibitor, delaying the metabolism of ACh and increasing the likelihood of ACh binding to the partially blocked receptor. Thus, administration of edrophonium to a myasthenic patient should increase the strength of involved muscles.

4. An eyelid may appear ptotic even when it is normal, if compared to a retracted eyelid (e.g., proptosis) on the opposite side. Likewise, a normal lid may look ptotic if the eyeball itself is retracted into the orbit due to loss of orbital tissue.

RIGIDITY

DOPAMINE

Dystonia
Olivopontocerebellar atrophy (OPCA)
Parkinson's
Ankylosing spondylitis
Meningismus (meningitis, subarachnoid hemorrhage)
Increased tone/spasticity
Neuroleptic malignant syndrome
Elevated intracranial pressure

Notes

Rigidity is a continuous or intermittent increase in muscle tone throughout the full range of passive movement.

- Cogwheeling is a form of rigidity characterized by rhythmic, rachet-like resistance throughout the range of motion.
- Lead-pipe is a form of rigidity characterized by uniform resistance throughout the range of motion.

Spasticity is an increase in muscle tone that is mild with slow movement and more pronounced with rapid movement. Classically, rapid passive movement is met with increasing resistance until a point at which the resistance breaks ("clasp knife phenomenon").

1. Rigidity may be caused by:
   a. Neurologic pathology
      - Extrapyramidal/basal ganglia disorders (dystonia, olivopontocerebellar atrophy, Parkinson's, drug effects)
      - Corticospinal involvement (spasticity, elevated intracranial pressure/herniation)
   b. Meningeal irritation (meningitis, subarachnoid hemorrhage)
   c. Skeletal immobility (ankylosing spondylitis, severe spinal osteoarthritis)

2. In general, increases in muscle tone may be due to **corticospinal** or **extrapyramidal** pathology. The term rigidity may be used to refer to hypertonus of extrapyramidal origin, and spasticity refers to increased tone of corticospinal origin. Distinguishing characteristics of each are summarized in the table. Extrapyramidal syndromes of rigidity are not usually associated with hyperreflexia, Babinski signs, or paralysis, and are more often associated with other movement disorders such as tremor, choreoathetosis, ataxia, and/or dystonia.

	Rigidity	Spasticity
	Cogwheel or lead-pipe	Clasp-knife
Associated abnormal movements	Yes	No
Associated weakness/paralysis	No	Yes
Deep tendon reflex/plantar response	Normal	Increased/upgoing

3. Acute generalized rigidity is often an emergent sign. Initial treatment aims at maintaining vital functions while rapidly determining the etiology.
   a. ABCs, vital signs, monitors, O_2
   b. Work-up by suspected diagnosis:
      - **Increased ICP/herniation:** EMERGENCY. May require intubation, hyperventilation, and/or mannitol. Diagnostic tests include head CT/MRI. Diagnostic considerations include mass lesion, intracranial bleed, CNS infection, head trauma.
      - **Meningitis:** EMERGENCY. Check CBC and differential, electrolytes, BUN/Cr, glucose, cultures, lumbar puncture (if no evidence of increased intracranial pressure).
      - **Subarachnoid hemorrhage:** EMERGENCY. Check CBC, platelets, PT/PTT (INR), electrolytes, BUN/Cr, glucose, head CT.

- **Neuroleptic malignant syndrome:** EMERGENCY. Rule out other causes of acute rigidity, obtain medication history, check tox screen, CBC, electrolytes, glucose, BUN/Cr.
- **Dystonia:** URGENT. Rule out other causes of acute rigidity, obtain medication history.
  c. Treatment is directed toward the underlying process.

4. Chronic rigidity is more likely a permanent sequelae of neurologic injury (spasticity) or a neurodegenerative condition (Parkinson's, OPCA), or due to skeletal limitations (ankylosing spondylitis, severe spinal osteoarthritis).

5. Acute iatrogenic dystonic reactions may occur in response to therapy with phenothiazines, haloperidol, antiemetics, and other related drugs. Treatment with diphenhydramine relieves the dystonia in most cases.

TREMOR

SHAKE IT UP

Stage fright/emotional
Hyperthyroid/hypoglycemia
Alcohol withdrawal
Kinesogenic
Essential/familial

Intention
Toxins/drugs/medications

Underlying metabolic conditions (uremia, hepatic encephalopathy, Wilson's)
Parkinson's

HELP, I'M SHAKING

Hypoglycemia
Essential
Lithium/valproate/other medications
Parkinson's

Intoxication (e.g., stimulants)
Metabolic/asterixis

Stage fright/emotional
Hyperthyroid
Alcohol withdrawal
Kinesogenic
Intention
Normal/physiologic
Genetic (e.g., Wilson's, Huntington's disease)

Notes

Tremor is defined as an involuntary rhythmic oscillatory movement.

Asterixis is a condition characterized by nonrhythmic, episodic loss of muscle tone. May be confused with tremor.

1. Tremor can be distinguished into three main types based on clinical features.

a. **Resting tremor** is typically a coarse, relatively slow (3–5 hertz) tremor that is maximal when the affected area is at rest. Usually associated with forms of parkinsonism.

b. **Intention tremor** is a rhythmic oscillation that becomes more pronounced as the affected area approaches a target, and is absent or minimal at rest and at the beginning of motion. Etiologies include all forms of cerebellar disease.

c. **Postural/action tremor** is a rhythmic tremor present when the affected area is actively maintained in a particular posture or during active movement, but absent at rest. Physiologic tremor, alcohol withdrawal, hyperthyroidism, and familial essential tremor are all good examples.

2. **Six cardinal signs of parkinsonism:** resting tremor, rigidity, bradykinesia, flexed posture, loss of postural reflexes, and "freezing." For a definite diagnosis of parkinsonism, at least 2 of the 6 features must be present, and at least 1 of the 2 must be either resting tremor or bradykinesia.

3. Parkinsonism may be divided into four major syndromes.

a. Idiopathic: No known etiology—Parkinson's disease.

b. Symptomatic: Due to an identifiable insult—drug-induced (phenothiazine, haloperidol), hydrocephalus, hypoxic, postencephalitic, parathyroid dysfunction, toxic (manganese, carbon monoxide, "designer" drugs—MPTP, cyanide), posttraumatic, tumor, infarction.

c. Parkinson-plus: Parkinsonian with additional significant symptoms—Alzheimer's disease, multiple system atrophy, progressive supranuclear palsy.

d. Genetic: Inherited forms of parkinsonism—Hallervorden-Spatz, Huntington's disease, Wilson's disease.

4. Intention tremor is characterized by impaired finger-nose-finger and heel-knee-shin maneuvers. These patients often have other evidence of cerebellar dysfunction, such as nystagmus and gait instability. Unilateral intention tremor is suggestive of focal cerebellar disease such as infarct, bleed, or tumor, and should be evaluated with MRI (CT if acute).

5. Postural or action tremor is not present at rest, and, although it is brought out by motor activity, is not greatly amplified upon approach to a target like intention tremor. Postural tremor may be obvious simply by holding the arms outstretched.

6. Two major types of action tremor include the following:

a. Physiologic: This tremor is simply an exaggeration of a normal phenomenon (usually 8–14 hertz). It is precipitated by many stimuli, including anxiety/fear, hyperthyroidism, caffeine, lithium, valproic acid, alcohol/drug withdrawal, exercise, and enhanced adrenergic stimulation (including pheochromocytoma).

b. Familial or essential tremor: Usually 4–8 hertz shaking of the hands or head, often able to be suppressed by alcohol, variable in intensity. If there is a family history (usually autosomal dominant), it is considered *familial tremor;* if family history is not evident, it is termed *essential tremor;* and if it manifests only late in life, it is called *senile tremor.*

7. Drugs associated with tremor include adrenergic drugs (albuterol, metaproterenol), stimulants (methylphenidate, cocaine, caffeine, amphetamine), theophylline, prednisone, valproic acid, and lithium.

8. Management of tremor depends upon the type of tremor.

a. Idiopathic parkinsonian tremor may respond to carbidopa/levodopa, dopamine agonists (bromocriptine, pergolide), or anticholinergics (trihexyphenidyl, benztropine).

b. Symptomatic parkinsonism also should be managed by treating the cause (i.e., discontinuing offending drug, identifying and eliminating toxin exposure, relief of hydrocephalus, etc.)

c. Severely disabling drug-resistant parkinsonian and essential tremors have been successfully treated with stereotactic thalamotomy.

d. Cerebellar tremor also may be treated depending on the cause (i.e., removal of hemorrhage, excision of tumor, etc.)

e. Essential tremor is effectively treated with either propranolol or primidone.

WEAKNESS*

MISS GIMP

Myelopathy (acute)/myopathy
Infection
Stroke
Systemic illness

Guillain-Barré syndrome
Iatrogenic/drugs
Myasthenia
Paralytic toxins/periodic paralysis

Note: MISS GIMP emphasizes the acute causes of motor weakness.

G, I'M LIMP, CAN'T STAND

Guillain-Barré syndrome

Iatrogenic (paralytic agents, aminoglycosides, steroids)
Myopathy/myositis

Lou Gehrig's disease (ALS, motor neuron disease—
  usually gradual)
Infection (polio, botulism)
Myelopathy (acute)
Periodic paralysis, porphyria, paraproteinemia

Cushing's
Arteritis/vasculitis/stroke
Neoplastic (meningitis, paraneoplastic)
Toxins (lead, arsenic, pufferfish, tick paralysis)

---

*Acute/subacute, bilateral with minimal sensory involvement

Systemic illness (anemia)
Thyroid
Addison's
Neuromuscular junction disease (myasthenia, Lambert-Eaton syndrome)
Diabetic amyotrophy

Notes

Weakness is the reported symptom or demonstrable sign of decreased strength of muscular contraction. The cause of weakness may be at any level of the motor unit (brain, spinal cord, nerve root, peripheral nerve, neuromuscular junction, or muscle). It also may occur secondary to systemic or psychiatric illness.

1. **Localization of weakness** can be determined from only a few qualities of the patient's complaints/physical signs: symmetry, sensory involvement, and deep tendon reflexes/plantar responses.

Lesion Location	Usually Symmetric	Prominent Sensory Loss	DTRs	Toes Up?
Central				
Brain	No	Often ipsilateral to weakness	Increased (decreased acutely)	Yes
Spinal Cord	Maybe	Yes, usually have sensory level	Increased (decreased acutely)	Yes
Peripheral				
Peripheral nerve	Maybe	Yes	Decreased	No
Neuromuscular junction	Yes	No	Decreased	No
Muscle	Yes	No	Decreased	No
Both				
Motor neuron disease	Maybe	No	Increased	Yes

DTRs = deep tendon reflexes
Muscle weakness due to brain lesions is discussed under "Stroke." Muscle weakness due to spinal cord lesions is discussed under "Myelopathy." Muscle weakness due to peripheral nerve lesions is discussed under "Neuropathy."

2. **Amyotrophic lateral sclerosis** (ALS; also called Lou Gehrig's disease, motor neuron disease) is unique in that it presents with chronic, progressive weakness,

and on examination has mixed upper (increased tone, increased DTRs, upgoing toes) and lower (atrophy, fasciculations) motor neuron signs.

3. Acute/subacute weakness can be an emergency, especially if the integrity of the airway and respiratory muscles is compromised. Diagnoses that merit careful monitoring of respiratory function include: Guillain-Barré, periodic paralysis, acute myelopathy (high cervical), and myasthenia. Serial vital capacities are critical in the management of these patients.

4. In general, *neuropathic causes of weakness* will be weaker distally and will have some sensory involvement, and neuromuscular junction and muscular causes of weakness will be weaker proximally and have no sensory involvement. In addition, *muscular causes of weakness* may show elevated muscle enzymes (CPK, aldolase).

5. **Guillain-Barré syndrome** is a singular neuropathic cause of acute/subacute weakness in which sensory complaints are not often prominent. It is characterized by symmetric, distal-to-proximal, progressive motor paralysis with areflexia. *Diagnosis* is often made clinically, but can be supported by delayed nerve conduction studies. Lumbar puncture may reveal elevated CSF protein without pleocytosis.

Treatment is either plasmapheresis or intravenous immunoglobulin. Careful monitoring of respiratory function (by **vital capacity**) and autonomic function (by vital signs) is necessary to determine when interventions such as intubation may be required. Other supportive care includes aspiration precautions (if not intubated), prophylaxis for deep venous thrombosis, decubitus prophylaxis, bowel and bladder care, nutritional supplementation, and range of motion exercises to prevent contractures.

6. **Myasthenia gravis** can present with acute/subacute weakness and respiratory insufficiency. Typical clinical characteristics include waxing and waning symmetric proximal extremity and bulbar (cranial nerve) weakness with no sensory loss. *Diagnosis* is suggested by the clinical picture, and can be supported by a positive **Tensilon test** (see the Ptosis section). EMG also shows a characteristic decremental response to repetitive stimulation. Chest imaging may demonstrate an associated thymoma. Acetylcholine receptor antibodies may be detected in the serum.

Treatment acutely involves supportive care much as outlined above (for Guillain-Barré) with careful monitoring of vital capacity and intubation when necessary. Plasmapheresis and anticholinesterase drugs (pyridostigmine, neostigmine) are useful acutely. Thymectomy is indicated in all cases of thymic tumor, and may help in many other cases because of non-neoplastic thymic hyperplasia. Corticosteroids and other immunosuppressants (azathioprine, cyclophosphamide) are used for long-term therapy.

7. Patients who undergo **iatrogenic paralysis** for management of a ventilator have been reported to remain paralyzed for a prolonged period of time (days to weeks) after discontinuation of the paralytic agent, in spite of the (normally) short half-lives of these agents. The likelihood of prolonged post-treatment paralysis appears to increase with longer duration of therapeutic paralysis and with the severity of other systemic illnesses (especially renal failure).

8. **Endocrinologic causes of weakness** include the following:

Thyroid	Thyrotoxic—gradually progressive, especially in thighs/pelvic muscles, normal CPK
	Thyrotoxic periodic paralysis—attacks of symmetric weakness, usually with low K
	Thyroid ophthalmopathy—exophthalmos and weakness of extraocular muscles
	Myasthenia gravis—associated with dysthyroidism (either hyper- or hypo-)
	Hypothyroidism—diffuse myalgias, stiffness, slowed contraction, and relaxation of muscles
Adrenal	Addison's—generalized weakness, fatigability, associated with electrolyte imbalance
	Cushing's—proximal weakness, also may be seen after corticosteroid treatment

9. Systemic causes of nonspecific weakness may be secondary to anemia, congestive heart failure, malnutrition, deconditioning, cancer, etc.

10. Several paralytic intoxications may lead to acute weakness and even respiratory collapse. These include botulism, tick paralysis, pufferfish ingestion, and paralytic shellfish poisoning.

Clinical Conditions or Diagnoses

DEMENTIA

DEMENTIA

Degenerative
Ethanol/toxins/drugs (chronic)
Multi-infarct
Endocrine/metabolic
Normal pressure hydrocephalus
Tumor/trauma
Infection
Alzheimer's

DEMENTIA MIND

Degenerative (Parkinson's, Pick's)
Ethanol
Multi-infarct
Endocrine (thyroid disease, Cushing's, Addison's)
Normal pressure hydrocephalus
Tumor
Infection (HIV, neurosyphilis)
Alzheimer's

Metals and other chronic intoxications
Injury (contusions, chronic subdurals)
Nutritional/metabolic (B12 deficiency, Korsakoff's)
Depression/psychiatric (pseudodementia)

Notes

Dementia is an acquired condition characterized by chronic deterioration of intellectual function and associated with impairment in at least three of the following areas: language, memory, visuospatial skills, personality, and cognition. It is *not* associated with an acute confusional state.

1. By definition, *it is not possible to make a clear diagnosis of dementia in a patient with an acute encephalopathy.* Only after the encephalopathy clears can the diagnosis of dementia be entertained.
2. **Standard work-up** for reversible causes of dementia includes CT/MRI (*normal pressure hydrocephalus, neoplasm, multi-infarct*), TSH (*dysthyroidism*), VDRL/RPR (*neurosyphilis*), B12, and folate. If the onset is subacute or rapidly progressive, an LP (*subacute* and *chronic infections*) should be strongly considered.
3. Dementia must be distinguished from a number of other conditions.
   a. **Aphasia:** This is purely an abnormality of language expression/comprehension. With aphasia, it may be difficult to determine that the patient has intact memory and intellectual function. Aphasia may be a part of dementia, but by itself is suggestive of focal cerebral pathology.
   b. **Depression/pseudodementia:** Severe depression may manifest as extreme psychomotor retardation. Patients with pseudodementia have a primary psychiatric disorder, and the symptoms resolve upon successful treatment of this disorder. They tend to answer "I don't know" to direct questions, and show no evidence of cortical dysfunction like aphasia. This is usually a diagnosis of

exclusion. It is important to realize that depression can accompany many dementing illnesses without being the cause of the dementia.

c. **Acute confusional state/delirium:** This is the most important disorder to distinguish from a dementia, because delirium requires *urgent* diagnosis and treatment of its underlying cause. Clinical features associated with delirium include a waxing and waning course, abrupt onset, underlying medical disease, and hallucinations. It is possible for a demented patient to become delirious (i.e., a patient with Alzheimer's disease develops a cystitis or pneumonia and becomes more confused), but the diagnosis of dementia cannot be made for the first time in a delirious patient.

MYELOPATHY

BAD STRAIN

Bleed/hemorrhage/arteriovenous malformation
Abscess, epidural
Demyelinating disease (multiple sclerosis)

Spondylosis/stenosis
Trauma
Radiation
Arterial occlusion/vasculitis/infarction
Infection
Neoplasm

IT'S SAVING THE CORD

Idiopathic
Toxic/iatrogenic (intrathecal chemotherapy)
Systemic lupus erythematosus

Spondylosis/stenosis (degenerative spine disease)
Arachnoiditis
Vascular/ischemia
Infection (transverse myelitis, syphilis, Pott's
  disease/tuberculosis)
Nutritional (B12 deficiency)
Genetic (Friedreich's ataxia)

Trauma
Hemorrhage/arteriovenous malformation
Epidural abscess

Congenital (tethered cord, Chiari malformation, syrinx)
Oncologic (primary spinal tumors, epidural and bony
  metastases, carcinomatous meningitis)
Radiation
Demyelination (multiple sclerosis)

Notes

Myelopathy is any pathologic process leading to spinal cord dysfunction.

1. Clinical signs of a myelopathy include weakness and sensory loss below the level of spinal cord injury.

2. Although the classic motor findings of a myelopathy are upper motor neuron signs (spasticity, hyperreflexia, upgoing toes), **upper motor neuron signs may be absent acutely**; that is, acute motor findings of a myelopathy are often a flaccid paralysis.

3. A classic sensory finding of spinal cord dysfunction is a **sensory level**, i.e., numbness or sensory loss on the trunk below a certain dermatome. This is invaluable in localizing the segment of cord involved.

4. Remember that the spinal cord ends at L1-L2. If the lower extremities show upper motor neuron signs, and the upper extremities are normal, image the thoracic and upper lumbar spine. If all four extremities are involved, image the cervical spine.

5. **Acute myelopathy is a neurologic emergency.** Imaging is urgent in all cases, and IV methylprednisolone should be administered in cases of myelopathy resulting from trauma or neoplasm. Definitive acute therapy may include surgical decompression/spine stabilization and, for neoplastic disease, radiation.

6. It is important to obtain any history of trauma, back/neck pain, pre-existing cancer, multiple sclerosis, bowel/bladder dysfunction, and previous radiation to the spine.

Neuropathy

Primarily Motor

A TAD LIMP

Amyotrophic lateral sclerosis

Toxin (hexane, dapsone)
Anti-GM 1 antibodies
Demyelination (Guillain-Barré, chronic inflammatory demyelination polyneuropathy [CIDP])

Lymphoma
Infection (polio, diphtheria, hepatitis, HIV)
Metal, heavy (lead)
Porphyria

Primarily Sensory

GET PAIN OR NUMB

Genetic
Endocrine
Toxic

Polyclonal/monoclonal antibodies
Amyloid
Infection
Nutritional

Occupational (carpal tunnel)
Radiation

Neoplasm/paraneoplastic
Uremia
Medication
Brachial neuritis

MIXED SENSORIMOTOR

WEAK AND TINGLE

Work-related/trauma
Elevated IgG (paraproteinemia)
Autoimmune vasculitis (polyarteritis, lupus)
Kidney failure/uremia

Alcohol
Nutritional
Demyelination (CIDP)

Toxin (mercury)
Infection (HIV, Lyme disease)
Neoplasm/paraneoplastic
Genetic
Liver disease
Endocrine (diabetes, thyroid)

Notes

Neuropathy is any disorder that affects primarily peripheral nerves and is manifested by symptoms of weakness or sensory disturbance or both. Some disorders can mimic neuropathies by causing similar symptoms, and are included in the differential diagnoses above, even though they involve more than just the peripheral nerves (ALS, brachial neuritis).

Paresthesia is a sensation of numbness or tingling.

Dysesthesia is an uncomfortable sensation of tingling, prickling or burning, often elicited by light (normally nonpainful) touch.

Hypesthesia/hypoesthesia is a sensation of numbness; diminished sensation.

1. Clinically, the diagnosis of neuropathy can be aided greatly by categorizing the symptoms in two ways. First, by type of neuropathic disturbance; that is, primarily sensory, mixed sensorimotor, or primarily motor. Second, categorize the neuropathy by its onset/duration: acute (hours/days), subacute (weeks/months), or chronic (months/years).

Categorizing Neuropathy Symptoms

Onset/ Duration	Type of Disturbance		
	Primarily Motor	*Mixed Sensorimotor*	*Primarily Sensory*
Acute	Guillain-Barré syndrome Poliomyelitis AIDS (Guillain-Barré-like) Neuromuscular blockade (myasthenia, drug-induced) Myopathy (periodic paralysis)	Arsenic	Herpes zoster
Subacute	Chronic inflammatory demyelinating neuropathy Toxins (hexanes, lead) Paraproteinemia Neuromuscular disease (myasthenia) Myopathy (polymyositis) Motor neuron disease (ALS)	Diabetes AIDS Uremia Alcohol-related Nutritional deficiency (e.g., B_1, B_{12}, B_6) Toxins (hexanes, arsenic) Medications Rheumatologic Sarcoid Vascular Paraneoplastic Paraproteinemia Hypothyroidism Leprosy Critical illness polyneuropathy	Amyloid Herpes zoster Lyme disease Medication Nutritional deficiency (e.g., B_{12}, B_6, E) Paraneoplastic Post-radiation therapy Vitamin B_6 toxicity
Chronic	Paraproteinemia Hereditary motor sensory neuropathy Neuromuscular disease (myasthenia) Myopathy (muscular dystrophy) Motor neuron disease (ALS, post-polio syndrome)	Diabetes AIDS Uremia Alcohol-related Nutritional deficiency (e.g., B_1, B_{12}, B_6) Toxins (hexanes, arsenic) Medications Rheumatologic Sarcoid Vascular Paraneoplastic	Amyloid Hereditary sensory neuropathy Herpes zoster Lyme disease Medications Nutritional deficiency (e.g., B_{12}, B_6, E) Post-radiation therapy

(Table continued on next page.)

Categorizing Neuropathy Symptoms (Continued)

Onset/ Duration	Type of Disturbance		
	Primarily Motor	*Mixed Sensorimotor*	*Primarily Sensory*
Chronic (cont.)		Paraproteinemia Hypothyroidism Leprosy Hereditary motor sensory neuropathy Critical illness polyneuropathy	

2. The differential diagnosis for a primarily motor neuropathy includes other conditions such as motor neuron disease, neuromuscular junction (NMJ) dysfunction, and myopathies. Neuroanatomic localization can be difficult. Generally, the motor neuropathies cause decreased reflexes, while motor neuron disease (ALS) has increased reflexes and upgoing toes. Neuropathies and ALS tend to cause distal weakness, while in NMJ diseases and myopathies, the weakness is more proximal.

Clues for the Differential Diagnosis

Signs	Disorder		
	Neuropathy	*Myopathy/NMJ Disease*	*Motor Neuron Disease/ALS*
Atrophy	Yes, if chronic	Yes, if chronic	Yes, always chronic
Reflexes	Hypoactive	Variable	Hyperactive
Plantar response	Down	Down	Up
Distribution of weakness	Distal	Proximal, bulbar	Distal, bulbar
Fasciculations	Yes, if chronic	No	Yes, always chronic
Sensory loss	Yes, sometimes small	No	No

3. Acute weakness may be due to cerebral, neuropathic, neuromuscular, and muscular disorders. For differential diagnosis of generalized acute/subacute weakness see Weakness, page 246. For acute focal weakness see Stroke, page 262.

4. Chronic weakness in the absence of sensory complaints merits workup for NMJ disease, ALS, and myopathy, in addition to the few primary motor neuropathies. Using the above chart, try to distinguish clinically where the pathology is. Workup depends on the neuroanatomic localization and may include EMG/NCV, cervical MRI, tensilon test, CPK, aldolase, ESR, vitamin B_{12}, and urine/serum protein electrophoresis.

5. Most **nonacute neuropathies** fall into the category of sensorimotor or primarily sensory. There is a massive differential diagnosis for this, and workup should be aimed at the most common and the most treatable neuropathies (not necessarily the same).

Diagnostic Tests	Diagnosis
Serum glucose, glucose tolerance test	Diabetic neuropathy
BUN, Cr	Uremic neuropathy
TSH	Hypothyroidism, hyperthyroidism
Liver enzymes	Hepatic disease
Vitamin B_{12}	B_{12} deficiency
HIV	AIDS
ESR, ANA, RF	Polyarteritis nodosa, lupus,
Urine/serum protein electrophoresis	RA, etc.
Anti-Hu, -Ri, -Yo; guiac, CXR,	Paraproteinemia
mammogram	Paraneoplastic neuropathy
RPR, VDRL	Syphilis
Lyme titers	Lyme disease
Vitamin E Level	Vitamin E deficiency
Growth hormone, pituitary CT/MRI	Acromegalic neuropathy

Be careful with the shotgun approach! Don't order every test at once! Decide clinically which diagnoses are likely and test for those first. If no diagnosis is made and symptoms persist or worsen, continue the workup methodically. Also, *don't forget to look for risk factors* for neuropathies (e.g., alcohol, toxin exposure, family history, known malignancy, medications, known medical condition, IV drug use).

6. *Specific* treatment of neuropathies is aimed at the underlying cause. In addition, *symptomatic* relief may be helpful in cases of painful neuropathy. Here are some suggested medications and their uses:

Amitriptyline, other TCAs (low-medium dose)	Chronic painful neuropathies
Gabapentin	Painful neuropathies, diabetic, post-zoster
Capsaicin (topical)	Diabetic, post-zoster
Phenytoin, carbamazepine	Trigeminal neuralgia
Aspirin, ibuprofen, naproxen	General nonnarcotic anti-inflammatories
Codeine, oxycodone	General narcotic analgesics

7. In addition to pharmacologic intervention, general supportive care may be beneficial, including: physical therapy, range of motion exercises, padding, skin care, orthotics, safety awareness.

8. Medications known to cause neuropathy include:

Drug	Type of Neuropathy	Comments
Isoniazid	Initially sensory, then mixed	Treat concomitantly with B_6
Ethionamide	Similar to isoniazid	
Hydralazine	Similar to isoniazid	
Nitrofurantoin	Initially sensory, then mixed	Especially in uremics
Disulfiram	Initially sensory, then mixed	
Vincristine	Initially sensory or mixed	Dose related
Cisplatin	Primarily sensory	Especially proprioception/vibration

(Table continued on next page)

Drug	Type of Neuropathy	Comments
Chloramphenicol	Mild sensory	Associated with optic neuropathy
Phenytoin	Mild mixed sensorimotor	Associated with chronic (years) use
Metronidazole	Similar to phenytoin	Associated with chronic (years) use
Amitriptyline	Similar to phenytoin	Associated with chronic (years) use
Dapsone	Primarily motor	
Amiodarone	Mixed sensorimotor	5% of patients after months
Neuromuscular blockers	Primarily motor	Prolonged ventilation/ICU
L-tryptophan	Mixed sensorimotor	Associated with impurities, results in eosinophilia-myalgia syndrome

9. **Focal neuropathies**, rather than a general problem with all peripheral nerves, involve individual peripheral nerves and often are caused by local compression. Common syndromes include:

a. **Carpal tunnel syndrome**   Clinical: pain/numbness in digits 1–4, worse at night, rare weakness, positive Tinel's and/or Phalen's sign. **Location: wrist.** Diagnosis: NCV slow through carpal tunnel; risk factors are repetitive motion, rheumatoid arthritis, acromegaly, hypothyroidism, amyloid. Treat: anti-inflammatory drugs, wrist splints, proper adjustment of workstation/posture. Surgery is sometimes necessary.

b. **Ulnar neuropathy**   Clinical: pain/numbness in digits 4–5, hand weakness, claw-hand deformity. Diagnosis: NCV slow along course of ulnar. **Locations: several, especially elbow.** Treat: symptomatic, surgery to relieve compression.

c. **Radial neuropathy**   Clinical: wrist drop, impaired sensation on back of hand. **Location: axilla or upper arm.** Diagnosis: NCV; causes include crutch in axilla, arm over back of chair or edge of bed ("Saturday Night Palsy"), humeral fracture, lead toxicity. Treat: underlying cause.

d. **Meralgia paresthetica**   Clinical: lateral thigh pain/numbness, purely sensory. **Location: inguinal ligament.** Diagnosis: clinical; risk factors are obesity, pregnancy, diabetes, tight/heavy workbelt/harness, backpacking. Treat: relieve compression. Benign.

e. **Peroneal palsy**   Clinical: weak dorsiflexion of foot, top of foot numbness, often weak foot eversion. **Location: head of fibula.** Diagnosis: clinical, NCV; risk factors are plaster cast, prolonged leg crossing while seated, tight knee boots, emaciation, fibula fracture, diabetes. Treat: underlying cause.

Seizure

BITE TONGUE

Bleed/hemorrhage
Infection
Trauma
Ethanol/drugs/toxins

Tumor
Oxygen lack/ischemia/hypoxia
Noncompliance (subtherapeutic meds)
Glucose lack/hypoglycemia
Uremia/metabolic
Eclampsia

I CONVULSE BIG TIME

Infection

Cocaine/drugs
Oxygen lack/ischemia/hypoxia
Neoplasm
Vascular malformation
Uremia
Lytes (hypoNa, hypoMg, hypoCa)
Sinus thrombosis
Ethanol withdrawal

Bleed/hemorrhage
Idiopathic
Glucose lack/hypoglycemia

Trauma
Inborn error of metabolism
Medications (too much, too little)
Eclampsia

Notes

A seizure is a clinical manifestation of excessive, abnormal synchronous activity of neurons in the cerebral cortex. It is usually transient, and manifestations include alterations of consciousness, involuntary movements, sudden loss of motor tone, and sensory disturbances (especially olfactory or gustatory).

Epilepsy is a term reserved for chronic, recurrent seizures. A *single seizure does not make a diagnosis of epilepsy.*

1. The description of the seizure is helpful in diagnosis and treatment. A good description of a seizure includes any premonitory symptoms reported by the patient, any focal motor activity noted during the seizure, whether the motor activity was rhythmic and synchronous, the presence and direction of eye deviation, respiratory pattern, whether the patient was able to respond to verbal stimulus, whether the patient bit his/her tongue or experienced incontinence, and the presence and duration of post-ictal confusion.

2. **Major types of seizures:**

   a. Absence—staring, blinking, very brief, precipitated by hyperventilation, onset in childhood, no post-ictal confusion.

   b. Generalized tonic-clonic—all four extremities stiffen initially (tonic), then undergo rhythmic contraction and relaxation (clonic); post-ictal confusion is always present (to some degree); may be associated with cyanosis, tongue biting, and incontinence. *May often start as a focal/partial seizure and be secondarily generalized, particularly in adults.*

   c. Simple partial—may be motor (focal motor twitching) or sensory (focal sensory disturbance), with no alteration in level of consciousness during episode, no post-ictal confusion. *May secondarily become generalized tonic-clonic.*

   d. Complex partial—alteration in consciousness, automatisms (lip-smacking, eye blinking, swallowing, picking at clothes), preceded by aura (unusual smell, taste). *May secondarily become generalized tonic-clonic.*

3. **Treatment by seizure type**

   a. Treatment of absence seizure is primarily with ethosuximide or valproic acid.

   b. Treatment of primarily generalized seizures is usually with valproic acid.

   c. Treatment of secondarily generalized seizures is primarily with carbamazepine, phenytoin, or valproic acid.

   d. Treatment of partial seizures (simple or complex) is primarily with carbamazepine, phenytoin, or valproic acid.

   Other medications used to treat epilepsy include chlorazepate, clonazepam, felbamate, gabapentin, phenobarbital, primidone, tiagabine, topiramate, and lamotrigine.

4. It is important to distinguish between seizure, syncope, and psychogenic seizure/pseudoseizures.

   a. **Syncope** is typically preceded by a lightheadedness, precipitated by postural change, results in a fall/collapse with loss of consciousness lasting only seconds, and has no post-ictal confusion. Occasionally, a few myoclonic twitches may accompany syncope. Syncope is usually precipitated by a vasovagal reaction, but is also associated with arrhythmia, orthostatic hypotension, low cardiac output, and aortic valve disease. See the Loss of Consciousness section.

b. A **generalized tonic-clonic seizure** may also present with a fall/collapse, but is associated with grunting or apnea, occasional cyanosis, tonic then clonic motor activity, sometimes tongue-biting and incontinence, and always post-ictal confusion (usually lasting 5 minutes or longer). The duration of a generalized seizure is usually longer than a syncopal event, lasting seconds to minutes.

c. **Pseudoseizures** may be difficult to distinguish from epileptic seizures; indeed, the two disorders frequently overlap. In general, pseudoseizures occur in the presence of observers, are not stereotypic, have no post-ictal confusion, and are not associated with self-injurious activity like falling or tongue-biting. Motor activity includes completely asynchronous limb movements, struggling against restraints or resisting eye opening, and repeated side-to-side head movements. None of these is diagnostic, but careful observation helps avoid placing these patients on anticonvulsants or increasing dosages unnecessarily.

5. *The most common cause of a seizure in a patient with a known seizure disorder is subtherapeutic medication.* This may be due to noncompliance (due to side effects or lack of understanding) or increased dosing requirements.

6. Indications for neuroimaging studies:
   a. New focal-onset seizure or seizure with residual focal neurologic deficit
   b. Status epilepticus of unknown etiology
   c. New-onset seizure (uncertain focality) without known precipitant
   d. Any second seizure (except typical absence) not previously imaged.

It is not necessary to re-image a patient with a known seizure disorder after a typical seizure (see number 5 above). It is not necessary to image a child with typical absence seizures.

7. Indications for lumbar puncture:
   a. Status epilepticus of unknown etiology
   b. Patients under suspicion for subarachnoid hemorrhage
   c. Patients under suspicion for CNS infection (meningitis, encephalitis)

8. For seizures secondary to alcohol withdrawal and metabolic abnormalities, anticonvulsants are always second-line treatment; first-line treatment is directed at the underlying process (i.e., treat withdrawal, correct electrolyte abnormalities, correct hypoglycemia, etc.)

9. **Generalized convulsive status epilepticus** means continuous generalized convulsions or repeated generalized convulsions without *full* recovery of mental status between seizures for a period lasting greater than 30 minutes.

Protocol for treatment (Note: Items 1–4 are generally done nearly simultaneously)
   1. Carefully observe seizure activity. ABCs. Supplemental O_2 if necessary.
   2. IV line with normal saline. Send blood for CBC, electrolytes, BUN, Ca, Mg, glucose, anticonvulsant levels. Send ABG. Send U/A, consider tox screen. ECG monitoring.
   3. Accucheck, then 100 mg thiamine, then 50 ml of 50% dextrose solution if indicated.

4. Lorazepam 2 mg IV. Do not exceed 2 mg/min. May repeat up to 0.1 mg/kg. Call neurologist.
5. Phenytoin (Fosphenytoin) 20 mg(PE)/kg IV. When using phenytoin, do not exceed 50 mg/min. When using Fosphenytoin, do not exceed 150 PE (phenytoin-equivalents)/min. Monitor ECG, respiration and blood pressure.
6. Phenytoin (Fosphenytoin) 5–10 mg(PE)/kg IV. Maximum rates per minute as described above. Maximum dose 30 mg(PE)/kg.
7. Consider intubation if not already intubated.
8. Phenobarbital 20 mg/kg IV. Do not exceed 100 mg/min.
9. Consider barbiturate coma (in consultation with neurologist).
10. Common drugs having interactions with anticonvulsants include erythromycin, H_2 blockers, isoniazid, methylphenidate, phenothiazines, warfarin, oral contraceptives, and other anticonvulsants. Drug interactions may result in increased or decreased anticonvulsant levels or altered efficacy of the concomitantly administered drug. In general, newer anticonvulsants have fewer drug-drug interactions.
11. A *rough* clinical guide to phenytoin levels:

0–10	No nystagmus
Above 10:	Gaze-evoked nystagmus
Above 20:	Gait ataxia
Above 30:	Limb ataxia
Above 40:	Stupor/confusion

STROKE

SAVED BRAIN

Substance abuse/drugs/medications
Altered coagulation/hypercoagulability
Vasculitis
Emboli
Dissection

Bleed/hemorrhage/AVM
Rare causes (e.g., migraine, iatrogenic)
Atherothrombosis
Infections
Neoplasm

DEAD HEADS

Drugs/medications
Elevated blood pressure
Arteritis/vasculitis
Decreased perfusion (cardiac arrest, hypotension)

Hemorrhage or **H**ypercoagulability
Embolism
Atherosclerosis
Dissection
Spasm (migraine)

Note: "DEAD HEADS" emphasizes the vascular causes of stroke.

CVAS, DO I CT THEM?

Cocaine/drugs
Vasculitis/collagen vascular disease
Atherothrombosis
Syphilis, tertiary/meningovascular

Dissection/dysplasia (fibromuscular)
Oral contraceptives

Intracranial bleed (aneurysm, AVM)

Cancer
Thrombosis, sinus

Trauma/herniation
Hematologic*/hypercoagulable**
Embolic (including paradoxical)
Migraine

DO SAVE THEM BRAINS

Dissection/dysplasia (fibromuscular)
Oral contraceptives

Sinus thrombosis, venous
Atherothrombosis
Vasculitis/collagen vascular disease
Embolism (including paradoxical)

Trauma/herniation
Hematologic*/hypercoagulable**
Exogenous toxins/drugs (e.g., cocaine)
Migraine

Bleed/AVM/aneurysm
Radiation
Angiography
Infections (neurosyphilis, meningitis)
Neoplastic (bleed, meningitis)
Systemic hypotension/shock

---

*Thrombocytosis, polycythemia, sickle cell anemia
**Protein C deficiency or resistance, protein S deficiency, antithrombin III deficiency, malignancy, anticardolipin antibody syndrome, factor V deficiency, homocystinuria

Notes

Stroke refers to the sudden onset of a focal neurologic deficit that does not resolve. The etiology of a stroke is generally vascular, either hemorrhagic or ischemic. The vascular event may be precipitated by a different underlying cause (infection, tumor, hereditary condition).

Transient ischemic attack (TIA) refers to the sudden onset of a focal neurologic deficit that resolves in 24 hours or less.

Reversible ischemic neurologic deficit (RIND) is a neurologic deficit that lasts longer than 1 day and less than 3 weeks; essentially, a mild stroke.

Hemiparesis refers to a weakness on one side of the body. **Hemiplegia** refers to paralysis of one side of the body.

Astereognosis is the inability to identify objects by touch only.

Agraphesthesia is the inability to identify letters/numbers traced on the skin without visual cues.

1. Types of stroke

   a. **Hemorrhagic**—refers to focal bleeding, usually into brain parenchyma. Associated with acute hypertension, coagulopathy, amyloid angiopathy, occasionally trauma.

   b. **Thrombotic**—refers to gradual occlusion of cerebral arteries by local plaques/thrombi. Associated with longstanding hypertension, diabetes, atherosclerosis.

   - **Small vessel/lacunar**—occlusion of microvessels, typically in deep gray matter and/or brainstem.
   - **Large vessel thrombosis**—may not hear carotid bruit with a low-grade or a very high-grade stenosis.

   c. **Embolic**—refers to a sudden occlusion of cerebral arteries by blood clots that originate elsewhere in the vascular system. May be artery-to-artery (carotid to middle cerebral, aortic to carotid or vertebrobasilar), cardiogenic (heart to brain), or paradoxical (venous system through atrial septal defect to arterial system to brain). Associated with cardiac arrhythmias (especially atrial fibrillation), right to left shunts, valvular heart disease.

2. **Hemorrhagic strokes** can effectively be diagnosed by a noncontrast head CT. *Presentation* is usually that of a very abrupt onset of neurologic deficit which may not fit well into the vascular patterns described below. Very large hemorrhagic strokes in the cerebrum could result in decreased mental status secondary to herniation; *posterior fossa hemorrhages may lead to a very rapid decrease in level of consciousness.*

   Etiology is most often hypertension. *Treatment* consists of gentle control of extreme hypertension, supportive care, and occasionally (especially in posterior fossa/cerebellar bleeds) surgical evacuation. Anticoagulation is contraindicated. *Prognosis* for functional recovery after hemorrhagic strokes is usually better than after ischemic (i.e., thrombotic or embolic) infarcts.

3. Several stroke syndromes have been described as **lacunar/small vessel thrombosis**; that is, involving small infarcts as a result of occlusion of tiny penetrating vessels. These *presentations* include the following clinical syndromes:

   a. **Pure hemisensory deficit** (contralateral to a thalamic infarct)
   b. **Pure hemiparesis** (contralateral to an internal capsule infarct)
   c. **Clumsy hand-dysarthria** (multiple localizations)
   d. **Ataxia/hemiparesis** (both contralateral to a pontine infarct)

Onset of symptoms may be stuttering, stepwise deterioration or may be one of gradually worsening TIAs. The typical distribution of a hemisensory deficit involves the face, arm, and leg equally, because the sensory fibers are closely compact in the thalamus, so even a small ischemic lesion will likely affect all. Likewise for **pure hemiparesis**, which should be relatively **equal in the face, arm, and leg**, as the corticospinal fibers are crowded closely in the internal capsule

   Etiology is most likely chronic hypertensive damage to small penetrating vessels. *Treatment* acutely consists of avoiding hypotension, using antiplatelet agents, and supportive care. Long-term treatment involves diminishing risk factors such as smoking, hypertension, hyperlipidemia, and diabetes. Anticoagulation is unproven. Tissue plasminogen activator (TPA) may be beneficial within the first 3 hours.

4. Large vessel thrombosis may *present* with gradually worsening (crescendo) TIAs or an abrupt onset of symptoms Usually symptoms occur in a vascular distribution as described below. Carotid occlusion may present with only middle cerebral artery infarction (due to collateral flow to the ipsilateral anterior cerebral from the anterior communicating artery). *Etiology* is usually an atherosclerotic plaque with local thrombus formation. *Treatment* acutely includes TPA, avoiding hypotension, and supportive care. Carotid endarterectomy is indicated for *symptomatic* stenosis of 70% or greater, often in the setting of TIAs. Emergent carotid endarterectomy is unproven. Anticoagulation is unproven. Carotid endarterectomy in the setting of complete carotid occlusion is generally not indicated.

5. Embolism classically *presents* with an abrupt neurological deficit that is maximal at onset. Symptoms occur in a vascular distribution as described below. The hemiparesis of middle cerebral artery (MCA) occlusion differs from that of lacunar disease in that MCA infarction causes **hemiparesis that is greater in the face and arm than the leg** and is usually associated with hemisensory loss in a similar distribution. *Etiology* is by occlusion of an artery by a blood clot from either another artery (e.g., carotid to middle cerebral), the heart (cardiogenic), or the venous system via a right to left shunt (paradoxical). *Treatment* acutely may involve TPA, followed by anticoagulation, especially in cases of atrial fibrillation and small cerebral infarcts. Acute anticoagulation in the setting of a very large cerebral infarction has an increased risk of precipitating hemorrhagic transformation.

6. Localization of large vessel disease (**thrombotic** or **embolic**)

a. Specific signs/symptoms

• **Anterior** (i.e., carotid artery)	Monocular visual loss Agraphesthesia Visual-spatial deficits	Hemineglect Aphasia Astereognosis
• **Posterior** (i.e., vertebral basilar arteries)	Diplopia Ataxia Vertigo Face signs/symptoms opposite arm/leg signs/symptoms	Nystagmus Bilateral signs/ symptoms Vomiting
• Either	Hemiparesis Dysarthria Visual field cut (usually PCA, but may be present with large MCA infarctions)	Hemisensory loss

b. Vascular syndromes

• **Anterior cerebral artery**	Contralateral	Leg weakness > face/arm Incontinence

• Middle cerebral artery	Contralateral	Face/arm weakness > leg
		Hemisensory deficit
		Hemianopsia
• Posterior cerebral artery	Contralateral	Hemianopsia
		Mild hemiparesis
		Hemisensory deficit
• Vertebral basilar arteries	Contralateral	Hemiparesis
	Ipsilateral	Hemisensory deficit
	May be bilateral	Cranial nerve palsy
		Possibly hemiataxia

7. **Standard workup for stroke** includes a head CT (hemorrhage), CBC (thrombocytosis, polycythemia), glucose (diabetes), and lipids (hyperlipidemia). Other blood tests which may be useful include PT/PTT (coagulopathy, inadequate anticoagulation), ESR (vasculitis), and VDRL/RPR (neurosyphilis). Carotid duplex should be done in cases of anterior circulation strokes and TIAs. Transcranial Doppler is helpful in evaluation of posterior circulation (vertebrobasilar insufficiency). Echocardiography is performed to rule out valvular lesions and atrial or ventricular thrombi in patients suspected of having an embolic infarct. Magnetic resonance angiography is a noninvasive method of visualizing all of the cranial vasculature (anterior and posterior circulation), and the resolution of MRA has greatly improved over the last few years.

8. In **young patients** (< 45 years old) or patients with no clear etiology, the work-up for stroke/cerebral infarction can be much more extensive and may include protein C, protein S, anticardiolipin antibody, antithrombin III, factor V, and homocysteine (hypercoagulable states), angiography (arterial dissection, fibromuscular dysplasia, aneurysm), MRI (tumor, AVM), urine drug screen (cocaine, amphetamines), LP (infection, inflammation/vasculitis), and transesophageal echo with bubble study (atrial septal defect with paradoxical embolism).

9. Recently, the use of TPA has been recommended in acute stroke. Consider it in patients who present to medical care within 3 hours of onset of neurological symptoms, have significant neurologic deficits, and have no evidence of intracranial hemorrhage.

Neurology Glossary

Agraphesthesia is the inability to identify letters/numbers traced on the skin without visual cues

Akathisia describes an involuntary restlessness and inability to sit still.

Altered mental status refers to any acute or subacute change in the level of consciousness, ranging from mild confusion to deep coma. Synonymous with delirium. Chronic problems such as dementia or mental retardation are not considered in this category.

Amaurosis fugax is the subjective complaint of transient visual loss in one eye, often described as a veil or shade coming over the eye.

Astereognosis is the inability to identify objects by touch only.

Asterixis is a condition characterized by nonrhythmic, episodic loss of muscle tone. May be confused with tremor.

Ataxia is the subjective complaint or objective finding of impaired coordination, usually manifested as an impairment of gait or dexterity in the absence of significant muscular weakness.

Autonomic disorders constitute a wide range of neurologic derangements which may manifest primarily through symptoms of autonomic dysfunction, including but not limited to orthostatic hypotension/syncope, cardiac arrhythmias, altered lacrimation, impaired temperature regulation, diaphoresis/anhidrosis, sexual dysfunction, and bowel/bladder problems.

AVM is the acronym for arteriovenous malformation; an abnormal tangle of blood vessels that can develop in the central nervous system.

Choreoathetosis is an involuntary movement disorder characterized by rapid, jerky, dancing-like movements (chorea) associated with or superimposed upon writhing, flowing, continuous movements (athetosis).

Clonus is an abrupt, unidirectional series of muscular contractions in response to a sudden stretch. Also used to describe repetitive, rhythmic muscle contractions seen in some types of seizures.

Cogwheeling is a form of rigidity characterized by rhythmic, rachet-like resistance throughout the range of motion.

CT is the acronym for computed tomography, a diagnostic neuroimaging test.

CVA is the acronym for cerebrovascular accident; refers to any acute cerebrovascular pathology, generally ischemia or hemorrhage.

Dementia is an acquired condition characterized by chronic deterioration of intellectual function and associated with impairment in at least three of the following areas: language, memory, visuospatial skills, personality, and cognition. It is *not* associated with an acute confusional state.

Diplopia is the subjective symptom of double vision.

Dizziness is a symptom with many meanings, but particularly used by patients to refer to feelings of faintness/lightheadedness, vertigo, and/or unsteadiness/disequilibrium.

Dysconjugate gaze is the objective examination finding of eye misalignment, which may or may not be associated with symptoms of diplopia.

Dysdiadochokinesis is an impairment of the ability to perform rapid alternating movements.

Dysesthesia is an uncomfortable sensation of tingling, prickling, or burning, often elicited by light (normally nonpainful) touch.

Dyskinesia is an abnormality of movement. This usually refers to excessive motor activity (L-dopa-induced dyskinesias, tardive dyskinesia), but also may reflect a severe generalized slowing of movement (parkinsonian bradykinesia).

Dysmetria is impairment in the normal acceleration and deceleration of directed movements. Usually evaluated by finger-nose-finger and heel-knee-shin tests.

Dystonia is a condition of impaired muscle tone, which usually is increased, persistent, and at an extreme of the range of motion for the affected area.

EMG is the acronym for electromyogram, a diagnostic test that examines the electrical properties of muscle tissue (analogous to the electrocardiogram for the heart).

Epilepsy is a term reserved for chronic recurrent seizures. A *single seizure does not make a diagnosis of epilepsy*.

Gegenhalten describes an inability to relax muscles subjected to passive movement. On examination, it feels as if patient is resisting the examiner's motions.

Headache is a general term used to describe any painful sensation involving the structures of the cranium, face, and/or neck.

Hemiparesis refers to weakness/partial paralysis on one side of the body.

Hemiplegia refers to complete paralysis of one side of the body.

Hypesthesia is a sensation of numbness; diminished sensation. Synonymous with hypoesthesia.

Intention tremor is an exaggerated oscillation of a limb most pronounced as it is approaching a target, and essentially absent at rest or at the beginning of a movement. Intention tremor is a manifestation of dysmetria.

Lead-pipe is a form of rigidity characterized by uniform resistance throughout the range of motion.

LP refers to lumbar puncture; also known as a spinal tap.

Monocular visual loss is either a subjective report of transient visual loss in one eye (as opposed to one visual field) or an objective finding of decreased visual acuity in one eye.

MRI is the acronym for magnetic resonance imaging, a diagnostic neuroimaging test with higher resolution than CT, but which takes longer and is generally more expensive.

Myelopathy is any pathologic process leading to spinal cord dysfunction.

Myoclonus refers to a sudden, nonrhythmic contraction or spasm of a muscle or group of muscles. Contractions generally are unidirectional, asynchronous, and asymmetric.

Nerve conduction study is a diagnostic test that looks at the electrical function of peripheral nerves and roots.

Neuropathy is any disorder which affects primarily peripheral nerves and is manifested by symptoms of weakness or sensory disturbance or both.

Paresthesia is a sensation of numbness or tingling.

Ptosis is a physical finding of one palpebral fissure being smaller than the other, i.e., a drooping eyelid.

Reversible ischemic neurologic deficit (RIND) is a neurologic deficit that lasts longer than 1 day and less than 3 weeks; essentially, a mild stroke.

Rigidity is a continuous or intermittent increase in muscle tone throughout the full range of passive movement.

Seizure is a clinical manifestation of excessive, abnormal, synchronous activity of neurons in the cerebral cortex. It usually is transient, and manifestations include alterations of consciousness, involuntary movements, sudden loss of motor tone, and sensory disturbances (especially olfactory or gustatory).

Spasticity is an increase in muscle tone that is mild with slow movement and more pronounced with rapid movement. Classically, rapid passive movement is met with increasing resistance until a point at which the resistance breaks (clasp knife phenomenon).

Stroke refers to the sudden onset of a focal neurologic deficit that does not resolve. The etiology of a stroke generally is vascular, either hemorrhagic or ischemic. The vascular event may be precipitated by a different underlying cause (e.g., infection, tumor, hereditary condition).

Syncope is defined as a transient loss of consciousness and postural tone due to impaired cerebral blood flow. Synonymous with fainting.

Tics are stereotypic, involuntary, repetitive spasmodic muscular contractions. Typically able to be suppressed briefly, only to break out with increased severity. Often appear purposeful or semipurposeful.

Titubation is a moderate-frequency head tremor, usually antero-posterior.

Torticollis is a form of focal dystonia involving persistent contraction of cervical muscles, leading to a head tilt.

Transient ischemic attack (TIA) refers to the sudden onset of a focal neurologic deficit that resolves in 24 hours or less.

Tremor is defined as an involuntary, rhythmic, oscillatory movement.

Weakness is the reported symptom or demonstrable sign of decreased strength of muscular contraction.

XII

APPENDIX

Acronym Dictionary

ABG	Arterial blood gas
ALS	Amyotrophic lateral sclerosis
ANA	Antinuclear antibody
ARDS	Adult respiratory distress syndrome
ATN	Acute tubular necrosis
AVM	Arteriovenous malformation
AVP	Arginine vasopressin
BOOP	Bronchiolitis obliterans-organizing pneumonia
BUN	Blood urea nitrogen
CIDP	Chronic idiopathic polyradiculopathy
COPD	Chronic obstructive pulmonary disease
CPK	Creatine phosphokinase
CVA	Cerebrovascular accident
CXR	Chest x-ray
DDX	Differential diagnosis
DKA	Diabetic ketoacidosis
DVT	Deep vein thrombosis
ECG	Electrocardiogram
EEG	Electroencephalogram
ESR	Erythrocyte sedimentation rate
GERD	Gastroesophageal reflux disease
GVHD	Graft versus host disease
ITP	Idiopathic thrombocytopenic purpura
IVF	Intervertebral foramen
LAM	Left atrial myxoma
LP	Lumbar puncture
MCA	Middle cerebral artery
MCV	Mean cell volume

MI	Myocardial infarction
MS	Multiple sclerosis
NCV	Nerve conduction velocity
PCA	Posterior cerebral artery
PIE	Postinfectious encephalomyelitis
PT	Prothrombin time
PTT	Partial thromboplastin time
RDW	Red blood cell distribution width index
RPR	Rapid plasma reagin
SIADH	Syndrome of inappropriate secretion of antidiuretic hormone
SLE	Systemic lupus erythematosus
TIA	Transient ischemic attack
TPN	Total parenteral nutrition
TSH	Thyroid-stimulating hormone
VDRL	Veneral disease research laboratory
VOD	Veno-occlusive disease